454

Veterinary Nurs
Self-Assessment Questions
and Answers

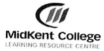

Senior commissioning editor: Mary Seager
Editorial assistant: Caroline Savage
Production controller: Anthony Read
Desk editor: Angela Davies
Cover designer: Helen Brockway

Veterinary Nursing:

Self-Assessment Questions and Answers

Second Edition

J. E. Ouston MA Vet MB MRCVS
Veterinary Surgeon and Lecturer in Veterinary Nursing
Farnborough College of Technology, Hampshire, UK

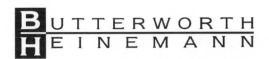

OXFORD   AUCKLAND   BOSTON   JOHANNESBURG
MELBOURNE   NEW DELHI

Butterworth-Heinemann
Linacre House, Jordan Hill, Oxford OX2 8DP
225 Wildwood Avenue, Woburn, MA 01801-2041
A division of Reed Educational and Professional Publishing Ltd

℞ A member of the Reed Elsevier plc group

First published 1997
Second edition 2000

British Library Cataloguing in Publication Data
Ouston, J. E.
    Veterinary nursing: self–assessment questions and answers.
    – 2nd ed.
    1. Veterinary nursing – Examinations, questions, etc.
    I. Title
    636' . 089' 073' 076

ISBN 0 7506 4803 1

Typeset by Latimer Trend and Company Ltd, Plymouth
Printed and bound in Great Britain by Biddles Ltd, Guildford and King's Lynn

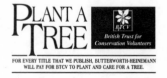

Contents

Contents

Preface

I wrote my first set of multiple choice books in 1996, and these proved to be very popular with trainee nurses, especially as a means of testing themselves prior to the Royal College of Veterinary Surgeons' examinations. In 1998 the syllabus was changed, and S/NVQs were introduced. I was asked to update my books to include the subjects that had been added, and to include other new developments in the veterinary profession.

The new book includes both S/NVQ level 2 and S/NVQ level 3 questions (the old Part I and Part II), and has been compiled to follow the chapter layout of *Veterinary Nursing* (2nd edition), edited by Lane and Cooper. However, there are a couple of differences I should point out. I have not included questions on behaviour problems or bereavement, since these are not subjects on which students will be examined by the RCVS, but I have added questions on human first aid, as this is now part of the students' syllabus. At the beginning of each subject I have given the number of questions to provide an indication of the amount of time that should be allowed. In the RCVS examinations, each paper consists of 90 questions and students have 90 minutes in which to complete it. Therefore, to practise examination technique, 1 minute should be allowed for each question. Each question is presented with four possible answers, from which the one correct answer has to be selected.

When answering multiple choice questions there are a few general tips that should be followed. Always read the question or opening statement carefully, checking for words like 'not' or 'untrue'. It is easy to lose marks simply by not reading the questions properly. If there are calculations in the section being covered, it may be best to do the other questions first and come back to the calculations. For many people they take longer than one minute, but since they carry no more marks than any other question it is important that not too much time is spent on these such that there is not enough time for the rest of the paper. It is also important not to rush the questions. Pace yourself, ensuring that you answer each question carefully but still allowing sufficient time for a final check of your answers.

The answers for all the questions can be found in a separate section at the end of the book. I have given explanations for the answers, in the hope that this book will also help you to understand the subjects more fully.

JEO
2000

Questions

1 Handling, control, observation and care of the patient

1. **If a hospitalized patient showed one of the following signs, which would give you cause for concern?**
   A Pink mucous membranes
   B A capillary refill time of 1–2 seconds
   C Slightly cloudy urine passed by a tom cat
   D Dark green vulval discharge in a bitch due to whelp without any straining

2. **What sign might you see to indicate an animal is in pain?**
   A Hypothermia
   B Icterus
   C Tachypnoea
   D Bradycardia

3. **The term that means straining is**
   A Haematuria
   B Dyschezia
   C Tenesmus
   D Epiphora

4. **Fatty faeces can be described as**
   A Diarrhoea
   B Dyschezia
   C Steatorrhoea
   D Faecal tenesmus

5. **Blepharospasm means**
   A A dislike of bright light
   B Screwing up the eyelids
   C Excessive tear production
   D Oedematous conjunctiva

6. **An animal showing which of the following signs would be described as showing epistaxis?**
   A   Repetitive vomiting
   B   Bleeding from ears
   C   Bleeding from nose
   D   Straining to pass faeces

7. **What is the normal temperature for a cat?**
   A   38.0–38.5 °C (100.4–101.6 °F)
   B   39–40 °C (102.2–104 °F)
   C   36–38 °C (98–101 °F)
   D   40–42 °C (104–107.6 °F)

8. **Haemoptysis means**
   A   Vomiting blood
   B   Blood in the anterior chamber of the eye
   C   Blood in coughed up sputum
   D   Blood in faeces

9. **After reduction of a dislocated hip, which of the following bandages would you apply to the hind limb of a dog?**
   A   Esmarch's bandage
   B   Ehmer sling
   C   Robert-Jones bandage
   D   Velpeau sling

10. **Tape muzzles could be used quite easily in all the following types of dogs except**
   A   Doliocephalic breeds
   B   Brachycephalic breeds
   C   Mesocephalic breeds
   D   Mesaticephalic breeds

11. **The vein most commonly used as a route for administering intravenous injections in the dog is the**
   A   Jugular
   B   Cephalic
   C   Sublingual
   D   Saphenous

12. The maximum volume of drug that should be administered to a large dog by intramuscular injection is
A   2 ml
B   3 ml
C   5 ml
D   10 ml

13. What temperature would it be appropriate for a hospital ward to be maintained at?
A   7°C
B   12°C
C   18°C
D   26°C

14. For which of the following conditions might it be appropriate to apply local heat?
A   Haemorrhage
B   Sprain
C   Sting
D   Abscess

The answers start on page   *113*

2 First aid

1. **Haemorrhage from the distal tail can be controlled by occluding which of the following arteries?**
   A   Coccygeal artery
   B   Femoral artery
   C   Aorta
   D   Brachial artery

2. **A dog is presented at the surgery with blepharospasm. Which of the following could cause this clinical sign?**
   A   Urinary infection
   B   Rectal tumour
   C   Ocular trauma
   D   Nasal foreign body

3. **Which wound is an example of a closed wound?**
   A   An abrasion
   B   A puncture wound
   C   A lacerated wound
   D   An aural haematoma

4. **If these animals were sitting in the waiting room of your practice, which would you consider had the most life-threatening condition, and should be seen first?**
   A   A cat that had been involved in a road accident with no apparent fractures, but with pale clammy mucous membranes, fast shallow respiration and subnormal temperature
   B   A dog with a fractured femur with normal capillary refill time and normal temperature
   C   An old cat in chronic renal failure that was drinking excessively
   D   A pup with a wasp sting on its nose

5. **The term used to describe a fracture in which the fragments have damaged other vital structures is**
   A   Compound fracture
   B   Comminuted fracture
   C   Complicated fracture
   D   Multiple fracture

6. **Splinting would be appropriate for which of the following fractures?**
   A   Fracture of the proximal humerus
   B   Scapular fracture
   C   Femoral head fracture
   D   Midshaft radius and ulna fractures

7. **Which statement regarding strains and sprains is correct?**
   A   A strain is an injury to a ligament within a joint caused by excess stress
   B   A sprain is an injury to a ligament within a joint caused by excess stress
   C   A sprain is an injury to a muscle or tendon caused by overstretching
   D   Strains and sprains are the same thing

8. **In cases of severe haemorrhage from a distal limb it may occasionally be necessary to apply a tourniquet. What is the maximum time a tourniquet can be left in place?**
   A   5 minutes
   B   10 minutes
   C   15 minutes
   D   20 minutes

9. **If you were presented with these patients, which would you treat first?**
   A   A pup that had chewed through an electric cable and was unconscious
   B   A cat that was vomiting acutely
   C   An old dog that had suffered a 'stroke' and was unable to balance or stand, and was very distressed
   D   A young dog with a severe wound to the back of the carpus that was bleeding profusely

10. **If you were performing cardiac massage on a large dog whose heart had stopped, how often should you apply compression?**
    A   20 times per minute
    B   40 times per minute
    C   80 times per minute
    D   120 times per minute

11. When is reactionary or intermediate haemorrhage seen?
A   At the time of injury
B   24–48 hours after the incident, while the vessel wall is undergoing repair
C   3 to 10 days after the original incident
D   None of the above

12. An owner calls the surgery to say that her hamster is distressed, and that there is something red protruding from under its tail. What advice do you give?
A   Keep the tissue moist using saline and bring the hamster straight down to the surgery
B   Apply slow gentle traction to the object – it should come free quite easily
C   There is no need to do anything – it will resolve spontaneously
D   Push the mass back, once inside the animal it should stay put

13. Which of the following conditions would you *always* advise an owner to bring to the surgery immediately?
A   Prolapsed eyeball
B   Bee sting
C   Vomiting animal
D   Bite wounds

14. The Heimlich manoeuvre is used for
A   Dislodging an oesophageal foreign body
B   Dislodging a tracheal foreign body
C   Dislodging a pharyngeal foreign body
D   Any of the above

15. Any lay person may administer first aid in an emergency. Which piece of legislation specifies this?
A   Animals Act 1971
B   Animal Health Act 1981
C   Protection of Cruelty to Animals Acts 1911–1964
D   Veterinary Surgeons Act 1966

16. You are out when you are stopped by someone whose dog has just been involved in a road traffic accident. The dog is still alive, is conscious, and its airway and breathing seem adequate. It is in shock. What can you do immediately?
A   Give the dog something to drink
B   Call a vet
C   Keep the dog warm
D   Give mouth to nose resuscitation

17. **The first thing you should do for an animal suffering from heat stroke is**
    A Call the veterinary surgeon
    B Cool it with cold water
    C Get it in the shade
    D Cover it in a blanket

18. **Which term describes the situation in which abdominal contents have escaped through a natural hole in the body wall to lie in a subcutaneous position, but can be pushed back through the hole into the abdomen?**
    A Strangulated hernia
    B Reducible rupture
    C Irreducible rupture
    D Reducible hernia

19. **In wound healing what do macrophages and monocytes do?**
    A Provide nutrients to the area
    B Clear cellular debris
    C Produce granulation tissue
    D Encourage wound contraction

20. **You should do all of the following as first aid treatment for an animal with a dislocated elbow except**
    A Confine the animal and encourage it to rest
    B Give cold compresses
    C Attempt to reduce the dislocation
    D Check airway, breathing and circulation

21. **An animal in shock may be given any of the following except**
    A Antibiotics
    B Oxygen
    C Intravenous fluids
    D Food and water

22. **Deep unconsciousness could be distinguished from death by checking**
    A Pupil size
    B Colour of the mucous membranes
    C Pedal reflexes
    D Muscle tone

23. **Subcutaneous emphysema is**
    A Fluid under the skin
    B Lymph under the skin
    C Pus under the skin
    D Air under the skin

24. Nystagmus can develop after which type of 'collapse'?
A   Shock
B   Electrocution
C   'Stroke-like' event
D   Anaemia

25. Signs of shock include all of the following except
A   Pale mucous membranes
B   Tachycardia
C   Increased body temperature
D   Weak pulse

The answers start on page   *116*

3 Poisons

8 Questions

1. **The specific antidote that can be given to an animal suspected of having been poisoned with organophosphates is**
   A   Sodium calcium edetate in saline solution
   B   Ethanol and sodium bicarbonate
   C   Atropine sulphate
   D   Acetyl cysteine

2. **Animals with ethylene glycol poisoning often develop which crystal within their urine?**
   A   Cystine
   B   Urate
   C   Calcium oxalate
   D   Struvite (ammonium triple phosphate)

3. **Paraquat poisoning leads to the development of which of the following clinical signs?**
   A   Polyuria and polydypsia
   B   Renal damage and respiratory distress
   C   Abnormal pigmentation of the hair
   D   Nervous signs

4. **The pesticide with an anaesthetic action, which causes a dramatic drop in body temperature and leads to hypothermia and death is**
   A   Sodium chlorate
   B   Paraquat
   C   Metaldehyde
   D   Alphachloralose

5. **If an animal is suspected to have been poisoned by paracetamol, which antidote can be used?**
   A   Sodium calcium edetate in saline solution
   B   Ethanol and sodium bicarbonate
   C   Atropine sulphate
   D   Acetyl cysteine

6. **Vomiting should not be induced in cases of which type of poisoning?**
   A   Ingestion of bleach
   B   Phenol ingestion
   C   Petroleum products ingestion
   D   All of the above

7. **For what purpose is warfarin used legally?**
   A   Insecticide
   B   Slugbait
   C   Rodenticide
   D   Herbicide

8. **Some poisons cause a change in haemoglobin which leads to a colour change in the animal's blood. Which of the following poisons does this?**
   A   Carbon monoxide
   B   Sodium chlorate
   C   Paracetamol
   D   All of the above

The answers start on page   *121*

4 Occupational hazards and human first aid

10 Questions

1. What is Special Waste, and how should it be disposed of?

A   This includes all waste contaminated with animal tissues, blood or excretions, and it should be collected in yellow plastic sacks and await collection and incineration by an authorized collector

B   This includes bodies of dead animals, which can either be incinerated by an authorized company or buried on the owner's property

C   This includes bottles and vials that are contaminated with drug products, and should be stored in yellow plastic bins until collected by an authorized collector

D   This includes all non-hazardous waste that can be collected as normal waste products

2. Which piece of legislation requires that employers make an assessment of the risks associated with the use of chemicals and drugs, and then provide ways of minimizing the danger to staff and public?

A   Health and Safety (First Aid) Regulations 1981

B   Reporting of Infectious Diseases and Dangerous Occurrences Regulations (RIDDOR) 1995

C   Controlled Waste Regulations 1992

D   Control of Substances Hazardous to Health (COSHH) Regulations 1988

3. In human first aid, for which of the following injuries would you use the Elevated Sling?

A   Fractured collar bone

B   Fractured wrist

C   Dislocated shoulder

D   Fractured upper arm

4. Which of the following would you NOT do for a person with severe haemorrhage from their leg?

A   Apply direct pressure

B   Apply a tourniquet

C   Elevate the limb

D   Lie the patient down

5. **You are alone with an adult who has collapsed for no obvious reason and is not breathing. What is your first course of action?**
   A   Start cardiac massage
   B   Start artificial respiration
   C   Call for an ambulance
   D   Start both cardiac massage and artificial respiration

6. **In human first aid, when performing cardiopulmonary resuscitation on an adult, how many breaths should you give and then how many compressions?**
   A   1 breath, 5 compressions
   B   1 breath, 10 compressions
   C   2 breaths, 10 compressions
   D   2 breaths, 15 compressions

7. **How long should the Accident Book be kept after the last entry?**
   A   1 year
   B   2 years
   C   3 years
   D   5 years

8. **If someone is suffering from shock, which of the following is appropriate treatment?**
   A   Persuade the patient to lie down and raise and support the legs
   B   Give the person a warm drink (not alcohol)
   C   Tell the patient to go and see his or her GP
   D   Shock is not serious, and therefore does not really need any treatment

9. **Burns are classified according to the area they affect and their depth through skin. Which of the following would you refer for further medical attention?**
   A   A partial thickness burn on a child
   B   A partial thickness burn on the arm of an adult
   C   A full thickness burn to the hand
   D   All of the above

10. **What is the RICE mnemonic used as an aid to remembering treatment for?**
   A   Fractures
   B   Shock
   C   Sprains
   D   Wounds

The answers start on page   *123*

5 Management of kennels and catteries

23 Questions

1. **For animals requiring quarantine, the period of isolation in the United Kingdom is**
    A   6 months
    B   9 months
    C   1 year
    D   Variable, depending on country of origin

2. **If the following animals were hospitalized at your surgery, which would you clean out first?**
    A   A bitch due to be speyed
    B   An old cat with renal failure
    C   A puppy with suspect parvovirus infection
    D   A dog with infected wounds

3. **The minimum temperature at which a kennel or cattery should be kept is**
    A   5°C
    B   7°C
    C   10°C
    D   12°C

4. **What is the minimum height of a dog kennel in a quarantine kennel?**
    A   1 m
    B   1.5 m
    C   1.8 m
    D   3 m

5. **Which of the following dogs is a member of the Toy Group?**
    A   Whippet
    B   Bichon Frise
    C   Lhasa Apso
    D   Dandie Dinmont Terrier

6. **To minimize the risk of respiratory infections, how many air changes per hour should take place in a kennel block?**
   A   At least 2
   B   At least 4
   C   At least 6
   D   At least 10

7. **All of the following statements about hypochlorites (bleaches) are true except**
   A   They are suitable for skin usage
   B   They are cheap
   C   They are good against fungi, bacteria and viruses
   D   They are suitable for use in food areas

8. **The disinfectant that is an example of a diguanide is**
   A   Formaldehyde
   B   Chlorhexidine
   C   Povidone-iodine
   D   Cetrimide

9. **How long should records of quarantined animals be kept after their release from quarantine?**
   A   At least 6 months
   B   At least 9 months
   C   At least 1 year
   D   At least 2 years

10. **A cat that is long-haired is the**
    A   Abyssinian
    B   Cornish Rex
    C   Ragdoll
    D   Scottish Fold

11. **After arrival in the UK, how long does an owner have to wait before being allowed to visit his or her own animal in quarantine?**
    A   1 week
    B   2 weeks
    C   1 month
    D   6 weeks

12. The disinfectant that is unsafe to use on skin is
   A   Chlorhexidine
   B   Cetrimide
   C   Glutaraldehyde
   D   Povidone-iodine

13. A styptic is something used to control slight haemorrhage, for example if the quick of a claw is accidentally cut. Which of the following can be used for this purpose?
   A   Friar's balsam
   B   Silver nitrate
   C   Ferric chloride
   D   All of the above

14. What is the definition of disinfection?
   A   The removal or destruction of micro-organisms but not necessarily bacterial spores
   B   The removal or destruction of all living micro-organisms including bacterial spores
   C   The removal or destruction of micro-organisms but not necessarily bacterial spores on skin or living tissue
   D   None of the above

15. The Basenji belongs to which group of dogs?
   A   Hounds
   B   Working dogs
   C   Utility breeds
   D   Gundogs

16. Animals in boarding kennels should be checked at least
   A   Every 2 hours
   B   Every 3 hours
   C   Every 4 hours
   D   Every 6 hours

17. Contaminated sharps, including needles and scalpel blades, should be disposed of in which of the following ways?
   A   They should be collected in a tough plastic bag and incinerated
   B   They can be disposed of with normal clinical waste
   C   They should be placed in purpose-made plastic containers with a hole too small to get a hand into, and then incinerated
   D   It does not matter – they can go into a normal landfill site

18. The design of a quarantine kennel must incorporate which feature?
A   Observation panels in doors
B   Double doors and gates to form 'traps'
C   Solid panels between kennels
D   All of the above

19. The type of disinfectant that is particularly toxic to cats is
A   Quaternary ammonium compounds
B   Chlorhexidine
C   Phenols
D   Povidone-iodine

20. Which cat has white socks on all four feet?
A   Burmese
B   Birman
C   Siamese
D   Abyssinian

21. What type of disinfectant, which also has detergent properties, inactivates phenol and hypochlorite disinfectants?
A   Quaternary ammonium compounds
B   Pine oil fluids
C   Chlorhexidine
D   Alcohol

22. The Act that provides detailed information about the necessary design and construction of a quarantine kennels is the
A   Animal Boarding Establishment Act 1963
B   Town and Country Planning Act 1971
C   Rabies Order 1974
D   Breeding of Dogs Act 1973

23. What are the requirements for an animal to be imported into the UK under the Pets Travel Scheme, which commenced in 2000?
A   It must be made totally identifiable by being microchipped
B   It must be vaccinated against rabies and blood tested to show that the vaccine has taken adequately
C   It must enter the UK only through specific routes
D   All of the above

The answers start on page   *125*

6 Practice organization, management, law and ethics

9 Questions

1. **Which of the following procedures would it be legal for a trainee veterinary nurse to undertake at the direction of his/her employer?**
   A   Cat castration
   B   Suturing a wound
   C   Descaling and polishing teeth
   D   None of the above

2. **What are the requirements of the Dangerous Dogs Act 1991?**
   A   Dogs of the specified breeds must not be bred, sold, exchanged or given away
   B   The dogs must be muzzled and on a lead at all times in a public place
   C   The dogs must be neutered, tattooed and identichipped
   D   All of the above

3. **If a client comes in to your surgery asking for a second opinion, who should you inform, if it has not already been done?**
   A   Your veterinary surgeon who will see the animal
   B   The owner's original veterinary surgeon
   C   The Veterinary Defence Society
   D   All of the above

4. **According to the RCVS, how long should client records be kept for after an animal has died, or a client has left the area?**
   A   1 year
   B   2 years
   C   4 years
   D   6 years

5. **'Dead files' is the term used to describe**
   A   Information that is no longer accessible
   B   Information that is out of date and inaccurate
   C   Information that pertains to animals which are dead
   D   Information that has been kept longer than is actually necessary

6. **Supersession arises**
   A   When a veterinary surgeon hands over a case to a second veterinary surgeon
   B   When a veterinary surgeon takes over a client from another veterinary surgeon without the latter's knowledge
   C   When a client is visiting two different veterinary practices for treatment
   D   When a client requests that they see another veterinary surgeon for the management of a particular case

7. **The Act that provides details about the practice of veterinary medicine and surgery in the United Kingdom is the**
   A   Protection of Animals Acts 1911–1988
   B   The Medicines Act 1968
   C   The Protection of Animals (Anaesthetics) Acts 1954 and 1964
   D   The Veterinary Surgeons Act 1966

8. **Which of the following is an offence under UK law?**
   A   To use a stray animal for scientific research
   B   To advertise a fight to be held between animals
   C   To cause suffering by failing to do something
   D   All of the above

9. **The Breeding of Dogs Act 1973 requires a person to license his or her premises if he/she**
   A   Owns more than four dogs
   B   Breeds from a bitch
   C   Keeps two bitches used for breeding and the pups are to be sold for profit
   D   Breeds particular breeds of dog

The answers start on page   *128*

7 Nutrition

12 Questions

1. **In cats, a deficiency of which nutrient can cause retinal degeneration?**
   A   Vitamin A
   B   Taurine
   C   Methionine
   D   Tryptophan

2. **The vitamin that affects the growth and mineralization of bones and increases calcium absorption from the intestine is**
   A   Vitamin A
   B   Thiamine
   C   Niacin
   D   Vitamin D

3. **The basal metabolic rate is**
   A   The amount of energy an active animal uses in a day
   B   The amount of energy a healthy animal doing nothing uses in a day
   C   The amount of energy needed to metabolize 1 kg of food
   D   The amount of energy released from 1 kg of food

4. **Unlike most species, guinea pigs require an adequate supply of which vitamin in their diet because they are unable to synthesize it?**
   A   Vitamin A
   B   Vitamin B
   C   Vitamin C
   D   Vitamin D

5. **A diet consisting solely of lean meat would be deficient in which nutrients?**
   A   Protein and fat
   B   Fat and B vitamins
   C   Calcium, phosphorus and fat-soluble vitamins
   D   Calcium, phosphorus and protein

6. **Which of the following is a good source of B vitamins?**
   A   Yeast
   B   Lean meat
   C   Green vegetables
   D   Cod-liver oil

7. **In growing animals, what ratio of calcium to phosphorus should be fed?**
   A   4 : 1
   B   3 : 1
   C   2 : 1
   D   1 : 1

8. **Which dietary imbalance could result in excessive bone proliferation, leading to the eventual fusion of vertebrae and limb bones?**
   A   Excess vitamin A
   B   Vitamin E deficiency
   C   Vitamin B deficiency
   D   Excess vitamin K

9. **Copper is needed within the body for**
   A   Bone production
   B   Thyroid hormone
   C   Haemoglobin synthesis
   D   Nerve and muscle function

10. **Increasing fibre in the diet may be beneficial for animals with**
   A   Colitis
   B   Pancreatitis
   C   Cardiac disease
   D   Acute enteritis

11. **Which disease condition requires a diet low in protein, high in B vitamins and with increased carbohydrate?**
   A   Diabetes mellitus
   B   Obesity
   C   Renal disease
   D   Malabsorption syndromes

12. **Which of the following are B vitamins?**
   A   Tryptophan and thiamine
   B   Thiamin and vitamin K
   C   Riboflavin and ascorbic acid
   D   Thiamin and pantothenic acid

The answers start on page   *130*

8 Genetics

12 Questions

1. Epistasis is the term used to describe
A   An error produced in new DNA resulting in the alteration of a gene
B   Two genes on the same chromosome that are inherited together
C   Alternative forms of a gene at the same gene locus
D   The phenotypic effect of one gene obscuring the effect of another gene

2. A sex-limited gene is
A   Found on the sex chromosomes
B   Related to sexual characteristics
C   Found on the autosomal chromosomes, but only expressed in animals of one sex
D   None of the above

3. The name given to the position of a gene on a chromosome is the
A   Gene locus
B   Allele
C   Centromere
D   Autosome

4. Which characteristic is true of mitosis, but not meiosis?
A   Four daughter cells are produced
B   The daughter cells are identical to each other
C   The daughter cells are not identical to the parent cell
D   Only the sex cells divide this way, to form the sperm and ova

5. An animal that has two identical alleles for a particular gene is described as being
A   Homozygous
B   Homologous
C   Heterozygous
D   Hemizygous

6. **Mendel was one of the first people to study genetics, and from his observations on pea plants deduced two laws. What does Mendel's Second Law state?**
   A   Each pair of genes separates independently from others
   B   Genes exist in pairs
   C   Genes retain their identity from one generation to the next
   D   Discrete units of inheritance exist (genes)

7. **If the gene for blue coat colouring is recessive to black and tan colouring in Dobermans, what colour would the pups be if two blue Dobermans were mated?**
   A   All black and tan
   B   All blue
   C   Half of each colouring
   D   Three-quarters black and tan and a quarter blue

8. **Inherited and congenital defects are not the same. Which of the following is an inherited but not a congenital defect?**
   A   Umbilical hernia
   B   Progressive Retinal Atrophy
   C   Collie Eye Anomaly
   D   Cleft palate

9. **How would you describe the type of breeding if a bitch is mated with a dog to which she is related, though not closely?**
   A   In breeding
   B   Out breeding
   C   Line breeding
   D   None of the above

10. **If the gene for tabby colouring is recessive to black colouring in cats, how could you tell what the genotype of a black cat is?**
    A   Mate the cat with another black cat
    B   Mate the cat with its parent
    C   Mate the cat with a tabby cat
    D   None of the above

11. **If two genes are said to be linked, what does this actually mean?**
    A   They are always inherited together
    B   They are often inherited together
    C   They are never inherited together
    D   They code for similar characteristics

12. Which term is used to define the genetic make-up of a particular animal?
A   Genotype
B   Phenotype
C   Dominant characteristic
D   Homozygous

The answers start on page   *133*

9 Exotic pets and wildlife

20 Questions

1. **The animal which has a gestation period of over 60 days, and young that are born with fur and eyes open, is the**
    A   Guinea pig
    B   Rat
    C   Hamster
    D   Gerbil

2. **Which of the following species have no pads on their feet?**
    A   Guinea pigs
    B   Mice
    C   Rats
    D   Rabbits

3. **Ferrets reach sexual maturity at what age?**
    A   4–5 weeks
    B   6–7 weeks
    C   8–10 weeks
    D   6–9 months

4. **The gestation period of the chinchilla is**
    A   20–22 days
    B   24–26 days
    C   60–72 days
    D   111 days

5. **Induced ovulators are animals that require mating in order for the ovum to be released. Which of the following species is an induced ovulator?**
    A   Rat
    B   Bitch
    C   Ferret
    D   Chinchilla

6. **How can budgerigars be sexed?**
    A   Colour of the cheeks
    B   Colour of the cere
    C   Presence of striations under the tail
    D   All of the above

7. **The normal temperature for a rabbit is**
   A   38–40°C (100.4–104°F)
   B   37.4°C (99.4°F)
   C   40–41°C (104–105.8°F)
   D   36°C (96.8°F)

8. **To which order of birds does the canary belong?**
   A   Galliformes
   B   Psittaciformes
   C   Strigiformes
   D   Passeriformes

9. **Guinea pigs should be housed at temperatures of**
   A   0–12°C
   B   5–15°C
   C   12–20°C
   D   16–26°C

10. **At what temperature is a tropical fish tank usually kept?**
    A   10–12°C
    B   12–15°C
    C   16–20°C
    D   21–29°C

11. **Which of the following animals is ectothermic?**
    A   Tortoise
    B   Budgerigar
    C   Rat
    D   Chinchilla

12. **The type of hamster that can be kept in pairs is the**
    A   Syrian hamster
    B   Golden hamster
    C   Dwarf hamster
    D   None of the above

13. **Which of the following can you pick up by the tail?**
    A   Gerbil
    B   Rat
    C   Hamster
    D   Mouse

14. **The best technique for the restraint of a guinea pig is to**
    A   Catch hold of the base of the tail, and using the other hand catch hold of the scruff and lift
    B   Grasp around the shoulders with a thumb under the jaw and support the hind legs
    C   Hold the tail base and ears
    D   Grasp a large handful of scruff, including the ears, and lift

15. **Rabbits can be calmed by using which of the following methods?**
    A   Scruff the rabbit and include the ears
    B   Turn the rabbit over onto its back
    C   Cover its eyes
    D   Any of the above

16. **Which of the following chelonia species are predominantly herbivorous?**
    A   Box tortoises
    B   Terrapin
    C   Turtles
    D   Mediterranean tortoises

17. **Which term is used to describe difficulty in sloughing of the skin seen in snakes and other reptiles?**
    A   Dyschezia
    B   Dysecdysis
    C   Stomatitis
    D   White spot

18. **Which of the following species may require vaccinations?**
    A   Ferrets
    B   Chipmunks
    C   Guinea pigs
    D   Parrots

19. **What term is used to describe a female guinea pig?**
    A   Jill
    B   Doe
    C   Pen
    D   Sow

20. Which of the following small mammals exhibits mainly nocturnal behaviour?

A   Mouse
B   Hamster
C   Rat
D   Gerbil

The answers start on page   *136*

10 Anatomy and physiology

Cells, tissues and cell chemistry

12 Questions

1. **In intracellular fluid**
    A   Sodium concentration is high, chloride and potassium are low
    B   Sodium and chloride concentrations are low, potassium is high
    C   Sodium concentration is low, potassium and chloride are high
    D   Sodium and potassium concentrations are high, chloride is low

2. **An example of an electrolyte is**
    A   Salt
    B   Glucose
    C   Starch
    D   Fat

3. **Organelles are discrete membrane-bound structures found within the cytoplasm of cells. Which organelles are responsible for protein synthesis?**
    A   Mitochondria
    B   Golgi apparatus
    C   Ribosomes
    D   Lysosomes

4. **If a cell is placed in a hypertonic solution of sodium chloride, what will happen?**
    A   Water will move into the cell by osmosis
    B   Water will move out of the cell by osmosis
    C   Sodium chloride will move into the cell
    D   There will be no net movement of water or sodium chloride into or out of the cell

5. **Meiosis is one type of cell division. Which cells divide this way?**
    A   Nerve cells
    B   Intestinal cells
    C   The sex cells that form the sperm and ova
    D   Muscle cells

6. **Iron is needed within the body for**
    A   Haemoglobin, the pigment in red blood cells
    B   Bones and teeth
    C   Normal nerve and muscle function
    D   Blood clotting

7. **The average quantity of fluid lost per day by a healthy animal is**
   A   20–30 ml/kg
   B   30–40 ml/kg
   C   40–60 ml/kg
   D   60–80 ml/kg

8. **Which organ contains transitional epithelium?**
   A   Bladder
   B   Oesophagus
   C   Skin
   D   Blood capillary walls

9. **The mediastinum is the space formed between the two pleural sacs. Which structures lie within the mediastinum?**
   A   Heart, aorta and vena cava
   B   Heart, aorta, vena cava and lungs
   C   Heart and oesophagus
   D   Heart, aorta, vena cava, azygos vein and oesophagus

10. **An anabolic reaction occurs when**
   A   A complex substance is broken down into simpler molecules with the release of energy
   B   A complex substance is broken down into simpler molecules and energy has to be used
   C   Simple substances combine to form more complex molecules with the release of energy
   D   Simple substances combine to form more complex molecules and energy has to be used

11. **Areolar tissue is another name sometimes used for**
   A   Dense connective tissue
   B   Loose connective tissue
   C   Solid connective tissue
   D   Fluid connective tissue

12. **Hyaline cartilage is found in which of the following parts of the body?**
   A   The pinna of the ear
   B   The intervertebral discs
   C   The articular surfaces of bones
   D   The epiglottis

The answers start on page   *139*

The skeletal system

1. **Which of the following is a sesamoid bone?**
   A   Carpal bone
   B   Vertebra
   C   Patella
   D   Phalanx

2. **New bone is synthesized by**
   A   Osteoblasts
   B   Osteocytes
   C   Chondrocytes
   D   Osteoclasts

3. **The epiphysis of a bone is**
   A   The midshaft of the bone
   B   The end of the bone
   C   The growth plate region of the bone
   D   A fracture of a long bone

4. **Which of the following bones forms by endochondral ossification?**
   A   Carpal bone
   B   Parietal bone
   C   Patella
   D   Os penis

5. **The carnassial teeth in the dog are the**
   A   First upper molars and first lower molars
   B   Fourth upper premolars and first lower molars
   C   First upper molars and fourth lower premolars
   D   Fourth upper premolars and fourth lower premolars

6. **The unpaired bone in the skull that surrounds the foramen magnum is called the**
   A   Occipital bone
   B   Tympanic bone
   C   Zygomatic bone
   D   Vomer

7. **In which joint would you find a meniscus?**
   A   Elbow
   B   Carpus
   C   Temporo-mandibular joint
   D   Tarsus

8. **Vertebrae from which region of the spine have short spinous processes and long transverse processes directed ventrally and cranially?**
   A   Cervical
   B   Thoracic
   C   Lumbar
   D   Sacral

9. **At what stage during gestation do foetal bones ossify?**
   A   2–3 weeks
   B   4–5 weeks
   C   6–7 weeks
   D   8–9 weeks

10. **How many thoracic vertebrae are there in the dog?**
    A   7
    B   9
    C   11
    D   13

11. **The glenoid cavity is found within the**
    A   Shoulder joint
    B   Elbow joint
    C   Hip joint
    D   Temporo-mandibular joint

12. **The cranial cruciate ligament is an important structure within the**
    A   Tarsus
    B   Stifle
    C   Elbow
    D   Shoulder

13. **The appendicular skeleton contains all of the following bones except the**
    A   Scapula
    B   Sacrum
    C   Ilium
    D   Pubis

14. **Joints can be classified into several different types. Which of the following is an example of an amphiarthrosis?**
    A   Skull sutures
    B   Stifle
    C   The articulations between a rib and the vertebra
    D   Intervertebral disc

15. **What is the name given to the holes formed by adjacent vertebrae through which the spinal nerves emerge?**
    A   Foramen magnum
    B   Nutrient foramina
    C   Intervertebral foramina
    D   Vertebral canal

16. **The bone that forms the point of the hock is called the**
    A   Os calcis
    B   Anconeal process
    C   Tibial tuberosity
    D   Patella

17. **What is the dental formula for an adult cat?**
    A   I 3/3, C 1/1, PM 4/4, M 2/3
    B   I 3/3, C 1/1, PM 3/2, M 1/1
    C   I 3/3, C 1/1, PM 3/3
    D   I 3/3, C 1/1, PM 3/2

The answers start on page   *142*

The muscular system

12 Questions

1. **Epaxial muscles are found**
   A Below the transverse processes of the vertebrae
   B Surrounding the abdomen
   C Above the transverse processes of the vertebrae
   D In the limbs

2. **Contraction of the gastrocnemius muscle causes**
   A Extension of the stifle and flexion of the hock
   B Flexion of the stifle and extension of the hock
   C Flexion of the hock and extension of the digits
   D Extension of the hock and flexion of the digits

3. **Which of the following are striated muscles?**
   A Cardiac muscle
   B Muscles within the intestinal wall
   C Arrector pili muscles
   D Palpebral muscles

4. **All of these statements about cardiac muscle are untrue except**
   A It does not require energy for contraction to take place
   B It undergoes spontaneous contractions
   C It requires nervous stimuli to start contractions
   D It is easily fatigued

5. **The aponeurosis in the ventral midline where the abdominal muscles fuse is called the**
   A Prepubic tendon
   B Inguinal ring
   C Linea alba
   D Rectus abdominis

6. **The prime protractor of the forelimb is**
   A Brachialis
   B Biceps brachii
   C Brachiocephalicus
   D Trapezius

7. **The caudal thigh muscles are often called the hamstrings. Which three muscles make up the hamstrings?**
   A   Pectineus, biceps femoris and semitendinosis
   B   Biceps femoris, semimembranosus and semitendinosis
   C   Quadriceps femoris, semimembranosus and semitendinosis
   D   Biceps femoris, semimembranosus and gastrocnemius

8. **The Achilles tendon is formed by the tendons of insertion of several muscles. Which of the following does not form part of this tendon?**
   A   Semitendinosis
   B   Anterior tibial
   C   Biceps femoris
   D   Superficial digital flexor

9. **In which muscle's tendon of insertion is the patella found?**
   A   Biceps femoris
   B   Biceps brachii
   C   Gastrocnemius
   D   Quadriceps femoris

10. **The muscle that has its origin on the thoracic vertebrae is**
    A   Trapezius
    B   Supraspinatus
    C   Infraspinatus
    D   Triceps brachii

11. **All of the following are intrinsic muscles of the forelimb except**
    A   Latissimus dorsi
    B   Brachialis
    C   Supraspinatus
    D   Triceps brachii

12. **The adductor of the hindlimb is**
    A   Pectineus
    B   Quadriceps femoris
    C   Semimembranosus
    D   Gastrocnemius

The answers start on page   *145*

The integument

8 Questions

1. **What type of glands are mammary glands?**
   A   Merocrine glands
   B   Modified apocrine glands
   C   Sebaceous glands
   D   Mixed sebaceous and apocrine glands

2. **Which of the following is not a function of skin?**
   A   Waterproofing
   B   Vitamin D activation
   C   Vitamin E metabolism
   D   Fat storage

3. **Of the structures found in the dermis, which actually originate from the epidermis?**
   A   Sebaceous glands
   B   Nerve endings
   C   Capillaries
   D   Connective tissue

4. **The cerumen glands are found in the ear canal. What type of glands are they?**
   A   Apocrine glands
   B   Merocrine glands
   C   Sebaceous glands
   D   Endocrine glands

5. **What type of epithelium forms the epidermis?**
   A   Columnar epithelium
   B   Transitional epithelium
   C   Mesothelium
   D   Stratified squamous epithelium

6. **The functions of hair include all of the following except**
   A   Temperature regulation
   B   Colour markings for defence or recognition
   C   Vitamin D activation
   D   Sensory purposes

7. The tissue that forms the 'quick' of a claw is the
- A   Epidermis
- B   Dermis
- C   Coronary band
- D   Digital vein

8. Where do epidermal cells divide within the epidermis?
- A   In the agranular or basal cell layer
- B   In the granular or parietal cell layer
- C   In the cornified or keratinized layer
- D   Epidermal cells divide in all of the cell layers

The answers start on page   *148*

The respiratory system

1. **Inspiration of air into the lungs is produced by contraction of the**
   A   Abdominal muscles
   B   Diaphragm
   C   Vertebral muscles
   D   Sternal muscles

2. **'Dead space' refers to which of the following when describing the respiratory tract?**
   A   Alveoli filled with fluid
   B   The last breath of a dying animal
   C   The tissue between the airways of the lungs
   D   The part of the respiratory tract that is not available for gaseous exchange

3. **The 'tidal volume' is**
   A   The maximum volume of air that can be inspired and expired in one breath
   B   The volume of air inspired and expired during normal respiration
   C   The volume of air left in the lungs after forced expiration
   D   The volume of air left in the lungs after normal expiration

4. **The order inspired air passes through the structures of the airways is:**
   A   Trachea, bronchi, alveolar ducts, respiratory bronchioles, alveoli
   B   Trachea, respiratory bronchioles, bronchi, alveolar ducts, alveoli
   C   Bronchi, trachea, respiratory bronchioles, alveolar ducts, alveoli
   D   Trachea, bronchi, respiratory bronchioles, alveolar ducts, alveoli

5. **Which statement is true?**
   A   The right lung has four lobes, the left lung has three lobes
   B   Both lungs have three lobes
   C   Both lungs have four lobes
   D   The left lung has four lobes, the right lung has three lobes

6. **Inspired air contains what percentage of oxygen?**
   A 5%
   B 10%
   C 21%
   D 79%

7. **The sinus connected to the nasal chambers, and lined with mucous membranes is the**
   A Maxillary sinus
   B Paranasal sinus
   C Mandibular sinus
   D Frontal sinus

8. **The term used to describe a fast respiratory rate is**
   A Tachypnoea
   B Tachycardia
   C Dyspnoea
   D Orthopnoea

9. **How does gaseous exchange across the alveolar walls take place?**
   A Osmosis
   B Diffusion
   C Active transport
   D Filtration

10. **Where are the respiratory centres in the nervous system?**
   A Hindbrain
   B Midbrain
   C Spinal cord
   D Forebrain

The answers start on page   *150*

Blood and the circulatory system

15 Questions

1. **The cellular component of blood produced from a megakaryocyte is the**
   A   Erythrocyte
   B   Lymphocyte
   C   Neutrophil
   D   Thrombocyte

2. **The innermost epithelial layer of the heart is called the**
   A   Endocardium
   B   Myocardium
   C   Pericardium
   D   Epicardium

3. **Which branch of the aorta supplies arterial blood to the head and neck?**
   A   Coeliac artery
   B   Cranial mesenteric artery
   C   Subclavian artery
   D   Common carotid artery

4. **All of the following are sites of lymphoid tissue except the**
   A   Spleen
   B   Lymph node
   C   Bone marrow
   D   Thymus

5. **White blood cells are divided into granulocytes and agranulocytes. Which cell is an agranulocyte?**
   A   Monocyte
   B   Neutrophil
   C   Eosinophil
   D   Basophil

6. **Deoxygenated blood in the systemic and pulmonary circulations is carried by which blood vessels?**
   A   Systemic arteries and pulmonary veins
   B   Systemic veins and pulmonary veins
   C   Systemic veins and pulmonary arteries
   D   Systemic arteries and pulmonary arteries

7. **Where are contractions initiated in the heart?**
   A   Atrio-ventricular node
   B   Bundles of His
   C   Sino-atrial node
   D   Purkinje fibres

8. **All these veins are paired except the**
   A   External jugular vein
   B   Saphenous vein
   C   Azygos vein
   D   Cephalic vein

9. **The name given to the caudal end of the thoracic duct which receives lymph from the hindlimbs, lumbar region and abdominal organs is the**
   A   Thymus
   B   Right lymphatic duct
   C   Tracheal duct
   D   Cisterna chyli

10. **Which blood vessel links the intestinal capillary bed with the capillaries within the liver?**
    A   Caudal vena cava
    B   Cranial mesenteric artery
    C   Hepatic vein
    D   Hepatic portal vein

11. **Phagocytosis of bacteria is carried out by which white blood cells?**
    A   Eosinophils
    B   Basophils
    C   Lymphocytes
    D   Neutrophils

12. **White blood cells can be differentiated from each other when stained using Romanowsky stains. Which white blood cell shows characteristic red granules throughout the cytoplasm after staining?**
    A   Neutrophil
    B   Eosinophil
    C   Basophil
    D   Monocyte

13. The name of the valve that separates the left atrium and left ventricle in the heart is the
- A   Tricuspid valve
- B   Mitral valve
- C   Pulmonic valve
- D   Aortic valve

14. Which lymph node can be palpated caudal to the stifle joint?
- A   Popliteal lymph node
- B   Accessory axillary lymph node
- C   Superficial inguinal lymph node
- D   Parotid lymph node

15. Antibodies are produced by
- A   Neutrophils
- B   Monocytes
- C   B-lymphocytes
- D   T-lymphocytes

The answers start on page   *152*

The digestive system

11 Questions

1. **All the following statements about bile are true except**
   A It contains enzymes to aid fat digestion
   B It contains pigments which are waste products of haemoglobin breakdown
   C It is produced by the liver
   D It contains bicarbonate and other electrolytes

2. **Which nutrient can be absorbed into the lacteals and enter the blood stream via the lymphatic system?**
   A Glucose
   B Fatty acids
   C Amino acids
   D Fibre

3. **Chyme is**
   A The mix of food, mucus and gastric secretions produced in the stomach
   B The milky fluid contained within the thoracic duct
   C The enzyme used to break down fats
   D The exocrine secretion produced by the pancreas

4. **The small intestine is divided into three sections. In which order does food pass through them after leaving the stomach?**
   A Duodenum, ileum, jejunum
   B Ileum, duodenum, jejunum
   C Jejunum, ileum, duodenum
   D Duodenum, jejunum, ileum

5. **In which part of the gastro-intestinal tract would you find villi?**
   A Stomach
   B Small intestine
   C Rectum
   D Colon

6. **The liver carries out all of the following functions except**
   A Deamination of protein breakdown products
   B Storage of iron
   C Storage of fat
   D Manufacture of proteins

7. **Which statement about the tongue is untrue?**
   A   It is involved in swallowing
   B   It is made of smooth muscle
   C   It carries sensory receptors for taste, texture, temperature and pain
   D   It can be used as an area for evaporation and heat loss

8. **The enzyme amylase is needed to digest which nutrient?**
   A   Fats
   B   Carbohydrates
   C   Proteins
   D   Vitamins

9. **Bile is released from the gall bladder under the action of which hormone?**
   A   Gastrin
   B   Secretin
   C   Pepsin
   D   Renin

10. **The region that is common to both the digestive tract and the respiratory tract is the**
   A   Pharynx
   B   Larynx
   C   Oesophagus
   D   Eustachian tube

11. **The fold of connecting peritoneum that links the stomach to the body wall is called the**
   A   Mesentery
   B   Ligament
   C   Parietal peritoneum
   D   Omentum

The answers start on page   *156*

The urinary system

10 Questions

1. **The area of the bladder where the ureters enter is called the**
   A   Trigone
   B   Apex
   C   Body
   D   Vertex

2. **Which statement is true concerning absorption and secretion in the renal tubule?**
   A   Glucose is reabsorbed in the distal convoluted tubule
   B   Some drugs are actively secreted into the proximal convoluted tubule
   C   Amino acids are secreted into the proximal convoluted tubule
   D   Hydrogen ions and bicarbonate ions are excreted regardless of the pH within the body tissues

3. **The function of the loop of Henle in the renal tubule is to**
   A   Excrete drugs
   B   Concentrate the urine
   C   Conserve or excrete ions for electrolyte balance within the body
   D   Excrete sodium and chloride ions to set up the concentration gradient between the cortex and the medulla of the kidney

4. **Filtration of blood by the kidney takes place in the**
   A   Glomerulus
   B   Proximal convoluted tubule
   C   Medulla
   D   Collecting duct

5. **The main function of the proximal convoluted tubule is**
   A   Reabsorption
   B   Potassium and sodium balance
   C   Concentration of the urine
   D   Formation of the concentration gradient through the medulla of the kidney

6. **Which of the following would you not normally find in urine?**
   A   Water
   B   Electrolytes
   C   Urea
   D   Protein

7. Aldosterone is a hormone that affects kidney function. Which of the following does it control?

   A   Water reabsorption by the kidney
   B   Potassium reabsorption in the distal convoluted tubule
   C   Sodium reabsorption in the distal convoluted tubule
   D   Drug excretion in the proximal convoluted tubule

8. What is the normal pH for canine urine?

   A   8
   B   7.5
   C   7
   D   6.5

9. The indentation in the side of the kidney where the renal artery and vein enter and leave the kidney is called the

   A   Cortex
   B   Hilus
   C   Pelvis
   D   Medulla

10. Anti-diuretic hormone acts on which part of the renal tubule?

   A   Proximal convoluted tubule
   B   Loop of Henle
   C   Collecting duct
   D   Glomerulus

The answers start on page   *158*

The reproductive system

1. **Testosterone is produced by which tissue in the male?**
   A   Interstitial cells (Cells of Leydig)
   B   Sertoli cells
   C   Spermatogenic cells
   D   Anterior pituitary

2. **In which order do the sperm pass through the following structures?**
   A   Urethra, epididymis, deferent duct, seminiferous tubules
   B   Seminiferous tubules, epididymis, deferent duct, urethra
   C   Seminiferous tubules, deferent duct, epididymis, urethra
   D   Epididymis, deferent duct, seminiferous tubules, urethra

3. **The part of the broad ligament called the mesometrium is**
   A   Associated with the ovary
   B   Associated with the uterine or Fallopian tube
   C   Associated with the uterus
   D   Not associated with any of the above

4. **The accessory gland(s) in the tom cat is(are) the**
   A   Prostate gland
   B   Anal glands
   C   Prostate and the bulbo-urethral glands
   D   Prostate, bulbo-urethral glands, anal glands, tail glands and scent glands

5. **An ovum travels through the female reproductive tract in which order?**
   A   Uterine tube, infundibulum, uterine horn, uterine body
   B   Infundibulum, uterine horn, uterine tube, uterine body
   C   Infundibulum, uterine tube, uterine body, uterine horn
   D   Infundibulum, uterine tube, uterine horn, uterine body

6. **The epididymis is**
   A   The site of sperm production
   B   Where the sperm are stored
   C   Where testosterone is produced
   D   Where nutrients for the sperm are produced

7. **The word used to describe a male animal in which only one testis descends is**
    A   Orchitis
    B   Monorchid
    C   Cryptorchid
    D   Sterile

8. **An animal that usually produces a litter of several young is described as being**
    A   Polyoestrous
    B   Multigravid
    C   Multiparous
    D   Primigravid

9. **The spermatic cord consists of which of the following structures?**
    A   Deferent duct
    B   Deferent duct, blood vessels and cremaster muscle
    C   Deferent duct, blood vessels, nerves and cremaster muscle
    D   Deferent duct, blood vessels, nerves, cremaster muscle and vaginal tunic

10. **Signs of proestrus in the bitch include all of the following except**
    A   Vulval swelling
    B   Bloody vulval discharge
    C   Courtship play
    D   Standing to be mounted

11. **The hormone responsible for the signs and the behaviour changes seen in oestrus is**
    A   Progesterone
    B   Oestrogen
    C   Follicle stimulating hormone
    D   Luteinizing hormone

12. **All of these statements about colostrum are true except**
    A   Colostrum is the first milk produced after parturition
    B   Colostrum contains more lactose than milk
    C   Colostrum contains more protein than milk
    D   Colostrum is important in the transfer of immunity to the offspring

13. How long (on average) is oestrus in the bitch?
A   3–5 days
B   7–10 days
C   12–15 days
D   24–30 days

14. The breeding pattern of the bitch is described in which of the following ways?
A   Induced ovulator; monoestrous
B   Induced ovulator; seasonally polyoestrous
C   Spontaneous ovulator; monoestrous
D   Spontaneous ovulator; seasonally polyoestrous

15. Which hormone do the developing Graafian follicles within the ovary produce?
A   Oestrogen
B   Progesterone
C   Luteinizing hormone
D   Follicle stimulating hormone

16. The placenta is formed from which layers surrounding the developing embryo?
A   Amnion and allantois
B   Allantois and chorion
C   Chorion and amnion
D   All three layers – amnion, allantois and chorion

17. Where is luteinizing hormone produced?
A   Anterior pituitary
B   Posterior pituitary
C   Hypothalamus
D   Adrenal glands

18. The term 'pseudocyesis' means
A   A benign tumour of the ovary
B   An animal that is neither male nor female, but has characteristics of both
C   False pregnancy
D   Menopause

19. Oestrus in the bitch can be detected using which of the following methods?
A   Monitoring behaviour to the male
B   Blood-testing for progesterone
C   Vaginal smears
D   Any of the above

20. An acrosome is found in the head of each sperm. It contains
A   Mitochondria to produce energy
B   Nutrients for the sperm
C   The nucleus
D   Enzymes to allow penetration of the ovum

The answers start on page   *160*

The nervous system

1. **What is myelin?**
   A   Dense connective tissue that surrounds bundles of neurones
   B   Loose connective tissue lying between neurones lying in a
       bundle
   C   Cell membranes of Schwann cells which wrap around the
       axons of most neurones
   D   None of the above

2. **Sympathetic neurones are carried by which spinal nerves?**
   A   Cervical and thoracic spinal nerves
   B   Thoracic and lumbar spinal nerves
   C   Lumbar and sacral spinal nerves
   D   Sacral and coccygeal spinal nerves

3. **Which cranial nerve supplies the thorax and abdomen with
   parasympathetic neurones?**
   A   Facial nerve VII
   B   Vestibulo-cochlear nerve VIII
   C   Glossopharyngeal nerve IX
   D   Vagus nerve X

4. **The parasympathetic nervous system is responsible for which
   of the following actions?**
   A   Dilation of the pupil
   B   Increased gut movement
   C   Raising the hair
   D   Increased heart rate

5. **The tissue layers that overlie the central nervous system are
   called the**
   A   Epidura
   B   Fat tissues
   C   Meninges
   D   Ramus

6. **Which statement is true about the withdrawal reflex?**
   A   It is a spinal reflex
   B   It is a cerebellar reflex
   C   It is a conditional reflex
   D   It is a complex reflex

7. **The cauda equina refers to**
   A   The nerves supplying the tail only
   B   The spinal nerves that supply the forelimb
   C   The spinal nerves that extend from the caudal end of the spinal cord and continue to run within the vertebral canal
   D   All the spinal nerves

8. **The third ventricle is found in which part of the central nervous system?**
   A   Forebrain
   B   Midbrain
   C   Hindbrain
   D   Spinal cord

9. **The part of the brain responsible for balance and co-ordination is the**
   A   Cerebral hemispheres
   B   Cerebellum
   C   Medulla oblongata
   D   Midbrain

10. **How do sympathetic neurones reach the head?**
   A   Via the sympathetic chain
   B   Via the cranial nerves
   C   They do not supply the head area at all
   D   Via the vagus

11. **What is a synapse?**
   A   The end of a neurone containing transmitter
   B   The junction between one neurone and another
   C   The cytoplasmic outgrowths that carry impulses towards the cell body
   D   The long cytoplasmic process which carries the nerve impulse away from the cell body

12. **The dorsal root of a spinal nerve consists of which types of neurones?**
   A   Somatic sensory and autonomic sensory neurones
   B   Somatic sensory and somatic motor neurones
   C   Autonomic sensory and autonomic motor neurones
   D   Somatic motor and autonomic motor neurones

13. Which area within the brain is responsible for special senses, memory and awareness, and voluntary control of movement?
   A   Cerebellum
   B   Cerebral hemispheres
   C   Medulla oblongata
   D   Midbrain

14. The dorsal root ganglion contains
   A   Cell bodies of all neurones
   B   Cell bodies of motor neurones
   C   Cell bodies of sensory neurones
   D   Cell bodies of autonomic neurones

15. Which cranial nerve is the trigeminal nerve?
   A   III
   B   IV
   C   V
   D   VII

The answers start on page   *164*

The special senses

10 Questions

1. **Information about taste is carried by which cranial nerves?**
   A V and VII
   B VII and IX
   C V and IX
   D X and XI

2. **What is pupil constriction called, and how is it produced?**
   A Miosis, parasympathetic contraction of circular smooth muscles
   B Mydriasis, parasympathetic contraction of circular smooth muscles
   C Miosis, sympathetic contraction of radial smooth muscles
   D Mydriasis, sympathetic contraction of radial smooth muscle

3. **Changes in final head position are detected by which of the following structures?**
   A Semicircular canals
   B Utricle and saccule
   C Cochlea
   D Middle ear

4. **The stapes bone is one of the ossicles found within the middle ear. Which membrane does it lean against?**
   A Round window
   B Oval window
   C Tympanic membrane
   D None of the above

5. **The uvea or uveal tract in the eye consists of the**
   A Sclera, retina and optic nerve
   B Cornea, aqueous humour, lens and vitreous humour
   C Ciliary body, iris and retina
   D Iris, ciliary body and choroid

6. Where is light refracted in the eye?
   A External surface of the cornea, anterior and posterior surfaces of the lens
   B External and internal surfaces of the cornea, anterior and posterior surfaces of the lens
   C Through the aqueous and vitreous humour
   D At the ciliary body and the retina

7. The Organ of Corti detects
   A Changes in head position
   B Head movement
   C Pressure
   D Different sounds

8. The sense of smell is carried by which cranial nerve?
   A I
   B II
   C VIII
   D X

9. Accommodation is the term used to describe the ability to focus. Which structure contains smooth muscles that enable an animal to accommodate for close and distant objects?
   A Ciliary body
   B Conjunctiva
   C Iris
   D Retina

10. The fluid found in the posterior compartment of the eye is
   A Lacrimal fluid
   B Aqueous humour
   C Choroid
   D Vitreous humour

The answers start on page *168*

The endocrine system

12 Questions

1. **The hormone produced by the posterior pituitary is**
   A   Adrenocorticotrophic hormone
   B   Calcitonin
   C   Luteinizing hormone
   D   Oxytocin

2. **The kidney helps control water balance within the body under the influence of**
   A   Adrenocorticotrophic hormone
   B   Anti-diuretic hormone
   C   Calcitonin
   D   Parathyroid hormone

3. **A hormone that does not affect the kidney is**
   A   Erythropoietin
   B   Aldosterone
   C   Anti-diuretic hormone
   D   All the above affect the kidney

4. **Which hormone causes peripheral vasoconstriction, tachycardia and pupil dilation?**
   A   Thyroid hormone
   B   Adrenaline
   C   Cortisol
   D   Insulin

5. **The brain contains which endocrine gland?**
   A   Hypothalamus
   B   Pituitary gland
   C   Thalamus
   D   Thyroid glands

6. **If calcium levels in the blood fall, which hormone is released?**
   A   Thyroid hormones
   B   Parathyroid hormone
   C   Vitamin D
   D   Calcitonin

7. **The hormone that regulates sodium levels in the body is**
   A   Angiotensin
   B   Cortisone
   C   Aldosterone
   D   Adrenaline

8. **Which of the sex hormones is formed by the interstitial cells in the testes?**
   A   Testosterone
   B   Oestrogen
   C   Interstitial cell stimulating hormone
   D   None of the above

9. **Adrenocorticotrophic hormone is released from the**
   A   Adrenal glands
   B   Anterior pituitary
   C   Parathyroid glands
   D   Posterior pituitary

10. **The adrenal glands are divided into two parts, the adrenal cortex and the adrenal medulla. Which hormone does the adrenal medulla produce?**
    A   Adrenaline
    B   Aldosterone
    C   Cortisol
    D   Adrenocorticotrophic hormone

11. **The thyroid hormones T_3 and T_4 are responsible for controlling which of the following?**
    A   Calcium balance
    B   Sodium balance
    C   Metabolic rate
    D   Stress reactions

12. **Which hormone stimulates gluconeogenesis by the liver?**
    A   Insulin
    B   Glycogen
    C   Glucagon
    D   Thyroid hormone

The answers start on page   *170*

11 Medicines: pharmacology, therapeutics and dispensing

15 Questions

1. **A product for external use should be dispensed in a**
   A Coloured fluted bottle
   B Plain glass bottle
   C Wide-mouthed jar
   D A child-proof pot

2. **Of the following drugs used topically in the eye, which causes pupil constriction?**
   A Miotics, e.g. pilocarpine
   B Mydriatics, e.g. atropine
   C Local anaesthetics, e.g. ophthaine
   D Hypromellose drops

3. **The dose rate for prednisolone is 0.5 mg/kg. How many 5 mg tablets would a 30 kg dog need?**
   A One
   B Three
   C Five
   D Two

4. **Which of the following contains antibodies to a toxin?**
   A Vaccine
   B Toxoid
   C Booster
   D Antitoxin

5. **Which piece of information is not *legally* required on the label of a dispensed medicine?**
   A Date
   B Name of drug and dosage
   C Owner's name
   D The words 'For animal treatment only'

6. **Which of the following drugs is an analgesic?**
   A Diazepam (Valium)
   B Doxapram (Dopram)
   C Buprenorphine (Vetergesic)
   D Atropine sulphate

7. The drug that is a Schedule 3 Controlled Drug is
A Diazepam
B Pethidine
C Cannabis
D Pentobarbitone

8. P products may legally be supplied by
A Anyone
B Pharmacists and veterinary surgeons
C Pharmacists, veterinary surgeons and some licensed saddlers and agricultural merchants
D Pharmacists, veterinary surgeons, saddlers, agricultural merchants and pet shops

9. Which class of drugs will suppress coughing?
A Anti-emetic
B Anthelminthic
C Antitussive
D Antibiotic

10. The abbreviation that means three times daily is
A bid
B po
C pr
D tid

11. The vet asks you to draw up an injection of dexamethasone for a cat that is suffering from an allergy to flea bites. The dose rate is 0.2 mg/kg. The cat weighs 5 kg, and the concentration of the drug is 2 mg/ml. How much should you draw up?
A 0.2 ml
B 0.5 ml
C 1 ml
D 2.5 ml

12. Which piece of legislation controls the supply, purchase and storage of Controlled Drugs?
A Medicines Act 1968
B COSHH regulations
C Health and Safety at Work Act
D Misuse of Drugs Act 1971

13. **A 5 kg dog is to be anaesthetized with thiopentone. The solution has been made up to 2.5%. The dose rate is 10 mg/kg. How many ml will be needed?**
    A   1 ml
    B   2 ml
    C   0.5 ml
    D   4 ml

14. **Why should POM and PML products not be stored in the consulting room?**
    A   They should always be kept in locked cupboards
    B   They should not be kept anywhere that members of the public have access to
    C   There is nothing wrong with them being kept in the consulting room
    D   Dispensing should be carried out where the client cannot see

15. **In a veterinary situation, which drugs should only be dispensed to animals under a veterinary surgeon's care?**
    A   P products
    B   POM products
    C   PML products
    D   All the above

The answers start on page   *173*

12   Laboratory diagnostic aids

27 Questions

1. **A centrifuge would be needed in order to carry out which of the following tests?**
   A   Measurement of packed cell volume (PCV)
   B   Haemoglobin estimation
   C   Red blood cell count
   D   Platelet count

2. **Dehydration is characterized by**
   A   Increased PCV and decreased plasma protein level
   B   Decreased PCV and decreased plasma protein level
   C   Decreased PCV and increased plasma protein level
   D   Increased PCV and increased plasma protein level

3. **Variation in erythrocyte size on a blood smear is called**
   A   Spherocytosis
   B   Poikilocytosis
   C   Anisocytosis
   D   Anisochromasia

4. **When present in urine, which substance can mask a positive glucose reaction on urine dipsticks?**
   A   Ketones
   B   Blood
   C   Penicillin
   D   Ascorbic acid

5. **A 10-year-old dog with chronic renal failure has a blood urea nitrogen of 90 mg/dl and a serum creatinine level of 4.0 mg/dl. The specific gravity of urine from this dog is most likely to be**
   A   Between 1.020 and 1.040
   B   Between 1.006 and 1.025
   C   Less than 1.006
   D   Between 1.030 and 1.055

6. **A cat is presented with pinpoint haemorrhages on the skin and mucous membranes. What is the most likely haematological abnormality?**
   A   Increased packed cell volume
   B   Decreased PCV
   C   Increased platelet count
   D   Decreased platelet count

7. **Severe parasitism can result in which of the following changes in the white blood cell picture?**
   A   Eosinophilia
   B   Neutrophilia
   C   Lymphocytosis
   D   Monocytosis

8. **The normal packed cell volume (PCV) for a cat expressed as a percentage is**
   A   10–15
   B   16–23
   C   24–45
   D   46–58

9. **A differential white blood cell count should be stained using which of the following?**
   A   Leishman's stain
   B   Gram's stain
   C   Lugol's iodine
   D   New methylene blue

10. **Where are urinary casts produced in the urinary tract?**
    A   Kidney tubules
    B   Ureter
    C   Bladder
    D   Urethra

11. **What is the normal red blood cell count for a dog?**
    A $6–18 \times 10^9/l$
    B $5.5–8.5 \times 10^9/l$
    C $5.5–8.5 \times 10^{12}/l$
    D $6–18 \times 10^{12}/l$

12. **The white blood cells that usually make up 5% of the differential count are**
    A   Neutrophils
    B   Basophils
    C   Lymphocytes
    D   Monocytes

13. **The reason white blood cell diluting fluid contains acetic acid is**
    A   To lyse the red blood cells
    B   To lyse the white blood cells
    C   To make the white blood cells more easily visible under the microscope
    D   To suspend the cells

14. **In order to determine a differential white blood cell count, what is the minimum number of white blood cells that should be counted?**
    A   50
    B   100
    C   200
    D   500

15. **The enzyme or biochemical parameter that gives most information about damage to liver cells is**
    A   ALT
    B   AST
    C   Cholesterol
    D   Bilirubin

16. **When examining faecal smears, which stain is used to identify undigested fats?**
    A   Alcoholic Sudan III
    B   Lugol's iodine
    C   Eosin
    D   New methylene blue

17. **Urine intended for bacterial studies should be preserved using**
    A   Toluene
    B   Formalin
    C   Thymol
    D   Boric acid

18. **If you had collected a urine sample by catheterizing a patient, which of the following would indicate clinical disease?**
    A Mucus
    B Spermatozoa
    C White cell casts
    D Transitional epithelial cells

19. **If you are staining a blood smear with Leishman's stain, how long should you leave the undiluted stain on the smear?**
    A 2 minutes
    B 5 minutes
    C 10 minutes
    D 20 minutes

20. **How is the total magnification of a microscope calculated?**
    A Eyepiece magnification + objective magnification
    B Eyepiece magnification × objective magnification
    C Eyepiece magnification ÷ objective magnification
    D Eyepiece magnification − objective magnification

21. **What does a colorimeter measure?**
    A The amount of light emitted by a coloured solution
    B The concentration of any substance in solution
    C The amount of light absorbed by a coloured solution
    D The different colours of light that will pass through a particular solution

22. **Before drawing off serum, a blood sample should be allowed to clot for at least**
    A 10 minutes
    B 30 minutes
    C 1 hour
    D 2 hours

23. **The bacterium that needs to be stained using the Ziehl–Neelsen staining technique is**
    A Clostridium tetani
    B Streptococcus
    C Salmonella
    D Mycobacterium tuberculosis

24. A supra-vital staining technique has to be used to identify which of the following cell types?

A   Red blood cells
B   Platelets
C   Neutrophils
D   Reticulocytes

25. Which abnormal constituent would you find in the urine of a dog suffering from obstructive jaundice?

A   Protein
B   Blood
C   Bilirubin
D   Fatty casts

26. The bacteria that would appear as Gram-negative rods under the light microscope are

A   Streptococci
B   Staphylococci
C   Clostridium tetani
D   Escherichia coli

27. Which urinary crystals are usually described as looking like 'coffin lids'?

A   Struvite (ammonium triple phosphate)
B   Urate
C   Cystine
D   Calcium oxalate

The answers start on page   *177*

13 Elementary microbiology and immunology

18 Questions

1. **The difference between Gram-negative and Gram-positive bacteria is**
   A   Gram-negative bacteria do not have flagella
   B   Gram-positive bacteria have an extra cell wall layer
   C   Gram-negative bacteria have an extra cell wall layer
   D   Gram-negative bacteria are not pathogenic

2. **Bacteria reproduce in which of the following ways?**
   A   Conjugation
   B   Spore formation
   C   Simple binary fission
   D   Mitosis

3. **Structural components of all viruses include**
   A   A capsule, cell wall and a cell membrane
   B   A cell wall, a cytoplasmic membrane and nucleic acid
   C   A protein capsid and nucleic acid
   D   An envelope, DNA, RNA and a cell wall

4. **The bacterium that can form spores is**
   A   Staphylococcus aureus
   B   Clostridium tetani
   C   Escherichia coli
   D   Bordetella bronchiseptica

5. **Which statement is true about exotoxins?**
   A   They are very heat stable
   B   They are not usually very toxic
   C   They are produced by Gram-positive bacteria
   D   They are only released when the bacterium dies

6. **The term 'commensal' is used to describe**
   A   Two or more bacteria producing infection at the same time
   B   A bacterium that requires the presence of another bacterium to cause disease
   C   Bacteria that are normally present in or on the host without causing damage
   D   Bacteria which are of benefit to the host

7. **Which term is used to describe curved bacteria?**
   A   Cocci
   B   Spirochaetes
   C   Bacilli
   D   Vibrios

8. **A selective medium provides growth factors that enhance the development of a particular bacterium and inhibit others. Which of the following is a selective medium?**
   A   Nutrient agar
   B   Chocolate agar
   C   Deoxycholate citrate agar
   D   Blood agar

9. **Anaerobic conditions are required to grow which type of bacteria?**
   A   Streptococci
   B   Escherichia coli
   C   Leptospira
   D   Clostridia

10. **What size (roughly) are viruses?**
   A   Nanometres, nm (1×10^{-9} m)
   B   Micrometres, μm (1×10^{-6} m)
   C   Picometres, pm (11×10^{-12} m)
   D   Millimetres, mm (1×10^{-3} m)

11. **The term 'facultative anaerobe' is used to describe**
   A   A bacterium that has an absolute requirement for oxygen
   B   A bacterium that grows optimally without oxygen
   C   A bacterium that can grow in the absence of oxygen but grows better when oxygen is present
   D   A bacterium that grows best in the presence of tiny quantities of oxygen

12. **What does a toxoid contain?**
   A   Antigen from a micro-organism
   B   Antibodies to a toxin
   C   Antigen from a toxin
   D   Antibodies to a micro-organism

13. Which of the following is true about dead vaccines?
A   Only one dose is needed for good protection
B   They are less long-lasting in effect than live vaccines
C   They are less safe than live vaccines
D   Most vaccines currently used are dead vaccines

14. Live attenuated vaccines should be stored at what temperature?
A $< +2°C$
B $+2$ to $+8°C$
C $+5$ to $+10°C$
D $+10$ to $+15°C$

15. Mature antibody-producing cells are called
A   Immunoblasts
B   T-cells
C   B-cells
D   Neutrophils

16. Animals are not routinely vaccinated before they reach 8–9 weeks of age because
A   Their immune system is too poorly developed to be able to respond
B   There may still be maternal antibodies within the plasma
C   There may still be maternal T- and B-cells within the plasma
D   The dose of the vaccine would be too great, and the animals would develop clinical signs

17. Which of the following cells are phagocytes?
A   Monocytes
B   Lymphocytes
C   Basophils
D   Eosinophils

18. An epidemic can be defined as
A   A disease normally present in an area
B   A disease that has suddenly increased in prevalence in an area
C   A sudden world-wide spread of disease
D   A sudden increase in a particular animal disease

The answers start on page   *183*

14 Elementary mycology and parasitology

1. **An example of a pathogenic yeast is**
   A   Aspergillus
   B   Trichophyton
   C   Candida
   D   Microsporum

2. **The type of medium used to culture fungi is**
   A   Selenite broth
   B   Sabouraud's medium
   C   McConkey agar
   D   Deoxycholate citrate agar

3. **A dog is presented at the surgery with alopecia around the eyes and muzzle without obvious pruritus. Which mite do you suspect?**
   A   Otodectes cynotis
   B   Demodex canis
   C   Sarcoptes scabiei
   D   Cheyletiella yasguri

4. **The larval stage of Toxocara canis that is infective is**
   A   Fourth-stage larvae (L_4)
   B   Third-stage larvae (L_3)
   C   Second-stage larvae (L_2)
   D   First-stage larvae (L_1)

5. **What is the proper name of the hookworm?**
   A   Uncinaria stenocephala
   B   Trichuris vulpis
   C   Toxascaris leonina
   D   Oslerus osleri

6. **Lice can be divided into two types, sucking and biting. Which of the following is a sucking louse?**
   A   Ctenocephalides felis
   B   Linognathus setosus
   C   Trichodectes canis
   D   Felicola subrostratus

7. **Trombicula autumnalis can cause clinical disease in some cats and dogs. Which stage of its life cycle is parasitic?**
   A   Larva
   B   Nymph
   C   Adult
   D   All of the above

8. **An intermediate host is always required by which of the following parasites?**
   A   Toxocara canis
   B   Toxoplasma gondii
   C   Toxascaris leonina
   D   Taenia hydatigena

9. **The parasite that typically causes intense pruritus and crusting of the ear tips is**
   A   Demodex canis
   B   Trichodectes canis
   C   Cheyletiella yasguri
   D   Sarcoptes scabiei

10. **You are performing faecal flotation on the faeces from a dog, and find a lemon shaped egg with a plug at each end. Which worm is the dog infested with?**
    A   Trichuris vulpis
    B   Uncinaria stenocephala
    C   Toxocara canis
    D   Toxascaris leonina

11. **The eggs of which parasite are glued to the hair shafts of its host?**
    A   Ctenocephalides felis
    B   Sarcoptes scabiei
    C   Otodectes cynotis
    D   Linognathus setosus

12. **Dermatophyte test medium (DTM) changes colour if fungi are cultured on its surface. What colour does it turn?**
    A   Orange
    B   Yellow
    C   Red
    D   Brown

13. **Toxoplasma can be transmitted from one host to another via all of the following routes except**
    A   Via meat from an intermediate host containing the organism
    B   Via the milk from queen to kitten
    C   Via food contaminated by cat faeces
    D   Via the placenta and afterbirths of aborted lambs

14. **The term that describes infestation by dipteran larvae is**
    A   Mydriasis
    B   Meiosis
    C   Myiasis
    D   Miosis

15. **The whipworm of dogs is**
    A   Aelurostrongylus abstrusus
    B   Oslerus osleri
    C   Trichuris vulpis
    D   Uncinaria stenocephala

16. **Pruritus and excessive epidermal scaling can be produced by which non-burrowing mite?**
    A   Cheyletiella
    B   Notoedres
    C   Sarcoptes
    D   Otodectes

17. **The parasite that reproduces asexually is**
    A   Toxocara cati
    B   Taenia hydatigena
    C   Ixodes ricinus
    D   Felicola subrostratus

18. **Visceral larva migrans in man is caused by which parasite?**
    A   Toxocara canis
    B   Toxascaris leoninum
    C   Toxoplasma gondii
    D   Echinococcus granulosus

19. **A paratenic host is best defined by which of the following statements?**
    A   The host in which a parasite has to undergo part of its life cycle, before it can reinfest the final host
    B   A host that carries an organism, and sheds it intermittently
    C   The animal in which the adult or reproductive phase of the parasite occurs
    D   A host that carries an immature parasite in its tissues. It has to be eaten by the final host for the parasite to complete its life cycle

20. Wood's lamp examination will cause which fungal species to fluoresce in some cases?

A   Trichophyton

B   Aspergillus

C   Microsporum

D   Candida

21. The stain used to examine fungi is

A   Gram's stain

B   Lactophenol cotton blue

C   Wright's stain

D   Iodine

The answers start on page   *187*

15 General nursing

10 Questions

1. **A decubitus ulcer is**
   A   A pressure sore
   B   Ulceration of the mucous membranes
   C   A very deep corneal ulcer
   D   The early stages of gangrene

2. **Higginson's syringe can be used for which of the following?**
   A   Flushing and irrigating the ear canal
   B   Delivering a specific fluid volume via a drip
   C   Giving an enema
   D   Drawing fluid from a chest or abdomen (thoracocentesis or paracentesis)

3. **You have been asked to collect equipment together to catheterize a cat. Which urinary catheter would you select?**
   A   Tieman's catheter
   B   Jackson's catheter
   C   Dowse's catheter
   D   Foley catheter

4. **If a patient had undergone oesophageal surgery, which method of forced feeding would be most appropriate?**
   A   Oro-gastric tube
   B   Gastrostomy tube
   C   Naso-gastric tube
   D   Pharyngostomy tube

5. **The owners of an elderly dog have asked you for some advice regarding its care. Which of the following would you suggest?**
   A   Restrict fluid availability
   B   Restrict protein in the diet and increase carbohydrate levels
   C   Increase energy levels within the diet
   D   To provide as much exercise as possible, particularly at weekends when the owners are around more

6. How large is 1 unit French Gauge?

A $\frac{1}{4}$ mm

B $\frac{1}{3}$ mm

C $\frac{1}{2}$ mm

D $\frac{3}{4}$ mm

7. A disease that is not associated with older age is
A   Osteoarthritis
B   Periodontal disease
C   Osteochondrosis
D   Diabetes mellitus

8. Dysphagia is
A   Difficulty swallowing
B   Difficulty eating
C   Difficulty breathing
D   Difficulty chewing

9. Prolonged recumbency can lead to several complications. Which is potentially the most serious?
A   Decubitus ulcers
B   Hypostatic pneumonia
C   Joint stiffness
D   Muscle wastage

10. Constipation in patients can be prevented by the use of
A   Low fibre diets
B   Kaolin
C   High fibre diets
D   None of the above

The answers start on page   *192*

16 Medical disorders: infectious diseases

19 Questions

1. **The cause of feline infectious anaemia is**
   A   Feline leukaemia virus
   B   Coronavirus
   C   Parvovirus
   D   Haemobartonella felis

2. **'Blue eye' is a complication encountered in dogs vaccinated with**
   A   Live canine distemper vaccine
   B   Inactivated canine adenovirus-1 vaccine
   C   Live canine adenovirus-1 vaccine
   D   Leptospira vaccine

3. **You test a 2-year-old clinically normal cat from a single-cat household for feline leukaemia virus infection with an in-house test kit. The result of the test is positive. What is the most appropriate advice for the owner?**
   A   Isolate the cat and retest in 3 months
   B   Euthanase the cat before it develops full-blown infection
   C   The result was probably inaccurate
   D   Isolate the cat, but do not bother to retest, as the second test is likely to be positive

4. **The incubation period for parvovirus in dogs is**
   A   2–3 days
   B   3–5 days
   C   5–7 days
   D   Over a week

5. **Which of the following organisms can become latent after an initial infection?**
   A   Feline parvovirus
   B   Canine adenovirus-1
   C   Feline herpes virus 1
   D   Bordetella bronchiseptica

6. **In samples of which bodily fluids might you find leptospira organisms in an infected animal?**
   A   Gut secretions and faeces
   B   Blood
   C   Urine
   D   Both blood and urine

7. **Chlamydia infection in a cat can be diagnosed using which diagnostic technique?**
   A   CITE test
   B   Microscopy of conjunctival scraping
   C   Haematology
   D   Microscopic examination of lacrimal fluid

8. **What is a fomite?**
   A   Another host that carries an organism in which the organism undergoes part of its life cycle
   B   An inanimate object that comes into contact with an infected animal, becomes contaminated, and then comes into contact with a non-infected animal
   C   Another host that carries the organism and can shed it at any time
   D   Another host that carries the organism and has to be eaten to pass on the infection

9. **Haemobartonella felis is thought to be carried by fleas. Which term best describes the way the fleas act as carriers?**
   A   Biological vector
   B   Intermediate host
   C   Transport host
   D   Paratenic host

10. **Which set of clinical signs most closely describes infection in the dog by Canine adenovirus-1?**
    A   Acute myocarditis or gastro-enteritis
    B   One of several syndromes including oculo-nasal discharges, pharyngitis, hyperkeratosis of pads and nose, nervous signs
    C   Acute pyrexia, petechial haemorrhages on gums, hepatic enlargement, possible neurological signs, collapse and death
    D   Dry hacking cough, retching, gagging and occasional serous nasal and ocular discharges

11. A disease that is zoonotic is
- A   Parvovirus
- B   Distemper
- C   Canine Hepatitis
- D   Leptospirosis

12. What is a saprophyte?
- A   An organism that lives on a larger organism and causes disease
- B   An organism that lives on dead organic matter
- C   An organism that benefits its host
- D   An organism that causes no harm nor good to its host

13. Viral diseases can be positively diagnosed in the live animal using which of the following methods?
- A   Histology
- B   Clinical signs
- C   Rising antibody titre
- D   A single measurement of serum antibody levels

14. All of the following statements are true about feline infectious peritonitis except
- A   The mode of transmission is not well understood
- B   It can produce two forms of the disease, a wet and a dry form
- C   The organism is resistant to many disinfectants, and can remain in the environment for long periods of time
- D   The fluid produced in the wet form is high in protein

15. Canine parvovirus is thought to have evolved from which other infectious virus?
- A   Canine distemper virus
- B   Feline influenza virus
- C   Feline panleucopaenia virus
- D   Canine herpes virus

16. The feline infectious agent that causes chronic stomatitis and gingivitis is
- A   Chlamydia psittaci
- B   Haemobartonella felis
- C   Feline calici virus
- D   Coronavirus

17. Which organism can last in the environment for up to a year?
A   Canine parvovirus
B   Canine distemper virus
C   Canine adenovirus
D   Leptospira icterohaemorrhagiae

18. For barrier nursing, all of the following statements are true except
A   Nurses should wear waterproof aprons, gloves and boots
B   They should treat isolated cases before the remainder of the in-patients
C   Animals in isolation should have their own sets of food bowls, cleaning utensils, grooming equipment and bedding
D   Animals with the same disease condition can be placed together in an isolation ward

19. If an unvaccinated cat is exposed to feline leukaemia virus for the first time, it is most likely to lead to persistent infection if the cat is
A   Over 4 months of age
B   6–8 weeks of age
C   Elderly
D   A neonate

The answers start on page   *195*

17 Medical disorders: non-infectious diseases

19 Questions

1. **For which of the following conditions would you advise a diet containing restricted levels of protein and sodium?**
   A   Colitis
   B   Feline urologic syndrome
   C   Food allergy
   D   Renal disease

2. **A hyperthyroid cat would show all of these clinical signs except**
   A   Bradycardia
   B   Weight loss
   C   Heat intolerance
   D   Mild diarrhoea

3. **A cardiac disease that is congenital is**
   A   Endocardiosis
   B   Cardiomyopathy
   C   Myocarditis
   D   Persistent right aortic arch

4. **The clinical sign that is not typically associated with small intestinal diarrhoea is**
   A   Tenesmus
   B   Weight loss
   C   Polyphagia
   D   Borborygmi

5. **A patient could develop keto-acidosis as a complication of which of the following conditions?**
   A   Diabetes insipidus
   B   Hyperthyroidism
   C   Hypothyroidism
   D   Diabetes mellitus

6. **An animal suffering from left-sided heart failure would show which of the following signs?**
    A   Ascites
    B   Right-sided cardiac enlargement
    C   Pulmonary oedema leading to a cough
    D   Jugular pulse

7. **Furunculosis is a severe example of which skin disease?**
    A   Pyoderma
    B   Seborrhoea
    C   Alopecia
    D   Hormonal disease

8. **The term orthopnoea is defined by which of the following?**
    A   Increased respiratory rate
    B   Decreased respiratory rate
    C   The animal assumes sternal recumbency with elbows abducted and breathes through its mouth
    D   The animal can only breathe lying stretched out on its side

9. **Which of the following dietary changes is most beneficial in patients with cardiac disease?**
    A   Increase protein
    B   Increase digestibility
    C   Decrease salt
    D   Increase carbohydrate

10. **Animals that are jaundiced show yellow discoloration of the mucous membranes and sclera. What can cause jaundice?**
    A   Excess red blood cell destruction
    B   Bile duct obstruction
    C   Liver disease
    D   All of the above

11. **Arterial blood pressure is at its maximum during which part of the cardiac cycle?**
    A   Atrial systole
    B   Atrial diastole
    C   Ventricular diastole
    D   Ventricular systole

12. What does isosthenuria mean?
A   The kidney produces a very weak urine
B   The kidney cannot dilute or concentrate the urine, so passes a urine similar in composition to protein-free plasma
C   Crystals within the urine
D   A decreased production of urine

13. Which bone condition is associated with chronic renal failure?
A   Marie's disease (chronic pulmonary osteoarthropathy)
B   Rubber jaw (secondary hyperparathyroidism)
C   Lion jaw (cranio-mandibular osteopathy)
D   Barlow's disease (metaphyseal osteopathy)

14. Food allergies can be diagnosed by
A   Intradermal testing
B   Restriction diets
C   Using antihistamines
D   All of the above

15. Calcium levels within the body are regulated by which hormones?
A   Thyroid hormones
B   Glucocorticoids and mineralocorticoids
C   Insulin and glucagon
D   Parathyroid hormone and calcitonin

16. The management of a fitting animal might include the use of which drug?
A   Phenyl propanolamine
B   Pentobarbitone
C   Prednisolone
D   Phenylbutazone

17. The hormone released by the kidney when blood pressure falls is
A   Erythropoietin
B   Aldosterone
C   Angiotensin
D   Renin

18. **Which cardiac disease causes the development of nodules on the cusps of the heart valves, which prevents them opening and closing normally, and is the most common cause of congestive heart failure in the dog?**
A   Endocarditis
B   Pericardial effusions
C   Endocardiosis
D   Myocarditis

19. **Increased serum amylase and lipase activities usually suggest**
A   Liver disease
B   Kidney disease
C   Intestinal disease
D   Pancreatic disease

The answers start on page   *200*

18 Obstetrics and paediatrics

23 Questions

1. **Oestrus can be prevented, suppressed or postponed by using which of the following types of drug?**
    A Oestrogens
    B Progestagens
    C Prostaglandins
    D Oxytocin

2. **If a lactating bitch was presented at the surgery showing signs of shivering, muscle spasm, collapse and disorientation, which post-parturient condition would you suspect?**
    A Metritis
    B Lactation tetani (eclampsia)
    C Mastitis
    D Parvovirus

3. **It is essential that neonates receive colostrum within 36 hours of birth or they will not receive the full value of the colostrum. Why is this?**
    A They cannot digest the proteins
    B They are unable to absorb the antibodies directly into the bloodstream
    C They lack the enzymes needed to break down the antibodies
    D The fat content is too high

4. **How long after birth do pups' and kittens' eyes open?**
    A 3–6 days
    B 7–9 days
    C 10–14 days
    D 15–21 days

5. **Which statement about the reproductive cycle of the queen is correct?**
    A She is seasonally monoestrous
    B She is non-seasonal
    C She is a spontaneous ovulator
    D None of the above

6. All of the following are types of foetal dystocia except
  A Foetal oversize
  B Breech presentation
  C Uterine inertia
  D Foetal monster

7. The puerperium is the term used to describe
  A The period immediately prior to parturition
  B The period after parturition during which the uterus returns to normal
  C The foetal membranes that are produced after all the foetuses have been born
  D The area immediately around the vulva

8. The hormone present through metoestrus in the bitch is
  A Oestrogen
  B Follicle stimulating hormone
  C Progesterone
  D Luteinizing hormone

9. In the event of a misalliance in the queen, which drug may be given to terminate the pregnancy?
  A Oestrodiol benzoate (Mesalin)
  B Megoestrol acetate (Ovarid)
  C Proligestone (Covinan)
  D None of the above

10. The average duration of oestrus in the bitch is
  A 4 days
  B 21 days
  C 18 days
  D 9 days

11. A breech birth occurs when a foetus is delivered in
  A Posterior longitudinal presentation, dorsal position, with head and legs extended
  B Anterior longitudinal presentation, ventral position, with head and legs extended
  C Anterior longitudinal presentation, dorsal position, with forelimbs and neck flexed
  D Posterior longitudinal presentation, dorsal position, with hindlimbs flexed

12. If an animal is primigravid it means that
   A   She has had a litter before
   B   She is only carrying one foetus
   C   This is her first litter
   D   The uterus is lying in an abnormal position

13. How often would you feed a week-old orphan pup that was being hand reared?
   A   Every 2 hours
   B   Every 4 hours
   C   Every 6 hours
   D   None of the above

14. Blood tests can be carried out to determine whether a bitch is ready to be mated or not. Which hormone is tested for?
   A   Luteinizing hormone
   B   Oestrogen
   C   Follicle stimulating hormone
   D   Progesterone

15. If a vaginal smear were taken from a bitch during oestrus, which cell type would predominate?
   A   Round epithelial cells
   B   Red blood cells
   C   White blood cells
   D   Cornified epithelial cells

16. What is strabismus?
   A   Straining to pass faeces
   B   A squint
   C   An inability to crawl
   D   A head tilt

17. Semen for artificial insemination (AI) is usually collected from the tom cat using which of the following methods?
   A   Electro-ejaculation
   B   Injection of testosterone
   C   Digital manipulation
   D   Artificial vagina

18. Vaginal smears can be stained using which of the following?
A   Leishman's stain
B   Wright's stain
C   Difquik
D   Any of the above

19. Which of the following species is an induced ovulator?
A   Dog
B   Cow
C   Ferret
D   Hamster

20. At what stage during pregnancy is palpation for pregnancy diagnosis possible?
A   1–2 weeks
B   3–4 weeks
C   5–6 weeks
D   Only after 6 weeks

21. During which stage in parturition are the foetal membranes passed?
A   First stage
B   Second stage
C   Third stage
D   Fourth stage

22. A whelping kennel should be maintained at
A   18°C
B   22°C
C   26°C
D   30°C

23. Which term is used for a developing pup once it is approximately 35 days old and has recognizable features?
A   Zygote
B   Embryo
C   Foetus
D   Conceptus

The answers start on page   *206*

19 General surgical nursing

20 Questions

1. **All of the following are laparotomy approaches except**
   A Pararectal
   B Paracostal
   C Sublumbar
   D Paracentesis

2. **After luxation and replacement of which joint would you use an Ehmer sling?**
   A Stifle
   B Elbow
   C Shoulder
   D Hip

3. **How long does Plaster of Paris take to reach full weight-bearing strength?**
   A 30 minutes
   B 2 hours
   C 12 hours
   D Longer than 12 hours

4. **A gastropexy might be indicated in the management of which condition?**
   A Gastric foreign body
   B Gastric neoplasia
   C Gastric torsion
   D Haemorrhagic gastro-enteritis

5. **Which of the following investigative techniques would provide most information about a lump that was suspected of being a tumour?**
   A Wedge biopsy
   B Needle biopsy
   C Needle aspirate
   D Exfoliative cytology

6. **The statement about glaucoma that is untrue is**
   A Drainage of aqueous humour is prevented
   B Glaucoma can be inherited
   C Intra-ocular pressure is decreased
   D Left untreated it can lead to permanent retinal damage

7. **In which of the following breeds would you find an increased incidence of tracheal collapse?**
   A Great Dane
   B Labrador
   C Cocker Spaniel
   D Yorkshire Terrier

8. **The condition that could be an indication for performing a urethrostomy in a male animal is**
   A Ruptured bladder
   B Hydronephrosis
   C Urethral calculi
   D Ectopic ureter

9. **What is orchidectomy?**
   A Surgical removal of one or both testes
   B Removal of a section of the vas deferens (deferent duct)
   C Surgical removal of the penis
   D Removal of a section of the urethra

10. **A transverse fracture of a long bone could be repaired using which of the following techniques?**
    A Cast
    B Plate
    C Intramedullary pin
    D Splint

11. **Animals with lymphosarcoma are most commonly treated using which type of tumour therapy?**
    A Chemotherapy
    B Radiotherapy
    C Surgery
    D Radioactive isotopes

12. **Fracture disease is the term used to describe**
    A Infection within the bone and bone marrow
    B Healing of a fracture where the bones are poorly aligned
    C Scar formation within muscle or joints after fracture healing has occurred which prevents normal use of the limb
    D Electrolysis of a bone due to implants of different metals being used together

13. **If you were on your own dealing with a suspected gastric torsion and had already called the veterinary surgeon, what would you do next?**
    A   Radiograph the abdomen
    B   Trocharize the abdomen using an 18G needle
    C   Attempt to pass a stomach tube
    D   Operate immediately

14. **All the following tumours affect bone and connective tissue. Which is benign?**
    A   Osteosarcoma
    B   Chondrosarcoma
    C   Osteochondroma
    D   Fibrosarcoma

15. **Which of the following is not a cardinal sign of inflammation?**
    A   Heat
    B   Swelling
    C   Cyanosis
    D   Pain

16. **Cataracts affect which part of the eye?**
    A   Aqueous humour
    B   Lens
    C   Cornea
    D   Retina

17. **Gangrene is**
    A   Formation of an abscess
    B   Mineralization and the deposition of calcium
    C   Sloughing of dead tissues
    D   Death of tissues, with or without bacterial invasion

18. **If an animal is suffering from keratitis, which part of the eye is inflamed?**
    A   Cornea
    B   Sclera
    C   Conjunctiva
    D   Eyelids

19. Which intramedullary pin is often used in pairs for the repair of epiphyseal fractures?

A   Steinmann pin
B   Rush pin
C   Kuntscher nail
D   Any of the above

20. A drain could be used in which of the following situations?

A   A shallow wound healing by second intention
B   A deep wound in which dead space has been produced by the surgical removal of some tissue
C   A small surgical wound healing by first intention
D   A cystotomy

The answers start on page   *211*

20 Theatre practice and care and maintenance of surgical instruments

29 Questions

1. **In order to move about in the operating room, how should scrubbed personnel pass each other?**
   A   Any way that is convenient
   B   Back to back
   C   Back to front
   D   Front to front

2. **To prepare a skin site for surgery, all of the following procedures are recommended except**
   A   Clip and then prepare the area three times using a surgical scrub solution and then alcohol
   B   Prepare the area centripetally, progressively moving toward the site of the incision
   C   Remove all clipped hair before beginning preparation of the site
   D   Remove all surface dirt before beginning the surgical scrub

3. **Sterilization cannot be achieved by**
   A   Boiling
   B   Autoclaving
   C   Infra-red radiation
   D   Ethylene oxide

4. **If you have scrubbed in order to assist with a surgical operation, in which order should you place the surgical drapes?**
   A   Closest to yourself first, and then proceeding in a clockwise direction
   B   Starting on the opposite side to yourself (the surgeon's side), and then proceeding in a clockwise direction
   C   Starting closest to yourself, then on the opposite side (the surgeon's side), and then the two ends
   D   Any of the above is acceptable

5. **Which statement is not true about hot air ovens?**
   A   Instruments sterilized in this way cannot be packaged
   B   The temperature does not need to be as high as for autoclaves
   C   Sharp instruments need 180 minutes at 150°C
   D   Mineral oil, waxes and petroleum jelly can be sterilized in
        this way

6. **Theatre design and management should allow for all of
   the following except**
   A   The minimum number of people should be allowed in
        theatre at any time
   B   The theatre should have two entrances
   C   The theatre should have an X-ray viewer
   D   The sinks and scrubbing-up area should not be in the
        operating theatre, but in a separate preparation area

7. **The holding time for sterilizing instruments for an autoclave
   operating at a pressure of 15 lb/sq. in (1.2 kg/cm^2) and a
   temperature of 121°C is**
   A   3 minutes
   B   10 minutes
   C   15 minutes
   D   30 minutes

8. **Surgical gloves are sterilized using which sterilization
   method?**
   A   Infra-red radiation
   B   Gamma radiation
   C   Ethylene oxide
   D   Autoclave

9. **Surgical procedures can be classified according to the degree
   of asepsis maintained during the operation. Which category
   would a cystotomy fit into?**
   A   Clean
   B   Clean-contaminated
   C   Contaminated
   D   Dirty

10. **The sterility monitor that responds to temperature and time
    only is the**
    A   Sterigauge
    B   TST strip
    C   Autoclave tape
    D   Browne's tube

11. **The suture material that remains the longest in a wound before it is broken down by enzymes is**
    A   Catgut
    B   Polyglycolic acid (Dexon)
    C   Polyglactin 910 (Vicryl)
    D   Polydioxanone (PDS)

12. **Assuming no complications, how long after surgery should skin sutures generally be removed?**
    A   2–3 days
    B   4–5 days
    C   7–10 days
    D   15–17 days

13. **In old nomenclature, what size suture material is one size thicker than 3/0?**
    A   2/0
    B   4/0
    C   1
    D   0

14. **Suture patterns are described as being apposing, inverting or everting. Which of the following suture patterns is an everting pattern?**
    A   Simple interrupted
    B   Horizontal mattress
    C   Cruciate mattress
    D   Ford interlocking suture

15. **Which is the smallest suture material size available?**
    A   0.2 metric
    B   6/0
    C   2 metric
    D   3/0

16. **The suture material that is monofilament is**
    A   Silk
    B   Catgut
    C   Polypropylene (Prolene)
    D   Polyglactin 910 (Vicryl)

17. If a curved cutting needle was examined in cross-section, how would it appear?
A   Triangular with the apex of the triangle on the inside of the curve
B   Triangular with the apex of the triangle on the outside of the curve
C   Square, with the corner on the inside of the curve
D   Round, with a fine, tapered point

18. How is wire suture material sized?
A   Gauge, e.g. 20 G
B   Metric, e.g. 6 metric
C   BPC gauge, e.g. 2/0
D   French gauge, e.g. 6 FG

19. The retractor that is not self-retaining is the
A   Langenbek retractor
B   Travers retractor
C   Gossett retractor
D   Gelpi retractor

20. ASIF cortical and cancellous bone screws can be distinguished in which of the following ways?
A   Cancellous screws are always fully threaded
B   Cancellous screws have tighter threads than cortical screws
C   Cortical screws have a hex screwdriver fitting
D   Cortical screws are more tightly threaded than cancellous screws

21. Jacob's chuck is used to position which orthopaedic implant?
A   Plate
B   Rush pin
C   Cerclage wire
D   Intramedullary pin

22. The needle holders that have scissors combined are
A   McPhail's needle holders
B   Bruce Clarke's needle holders
C   Olsen–Hegar needle holders
D   Mayo–Hegar needle holders

23. **The pilot hole for a 3.5 mm ASIF cortical screw should be drilled using which sized drill bit?**
    A   1.5 mm
    B   2.0 mm
    C   2.5 mm
    D   3.5 mm

24. **The forceps that have a rat tooth end are**
    A   Lane's forceps
    B   Bendover forceps
    C   Spey forceps
    D   Allis tissue forceps

25. **How should instruments be passed to a surgeon?**
    A   Ratchet open, rings first
    B   Ratchet open, tips first
    C   Ratchet closed, rings first
    D   Ratchet closed, tips first

26. **Strabismus scissors are used in which particular type of surgery?**
    A   Orthopaedic surgery
    B   Aural surgery
    C   Ophthalmic surgery
    D   General surgery

27. **The instrument that can be used as a haemostat is**
    A   Halstead mosquito forceps
    B   Allis tissue forceps
    C   Adson dissecting forceps
    D   Cheatle forceps

28. **Which blade is known as a tenotomy blade?**
    A   No. 10
    B   No. 15
    C   No. 11
    D   No. 20

29. **If liquid nitrogen is being used for cryotherapy, what minimum temperature is reached?**
    A $-20°C$
    B $-40°C$
    C $-100°C$
    D $-150°C$

The answers start on page   *216*

21 Fluid therapy and shock

14 Questions

1. **A 12.5 kg mongrel has been vomiting for 3 days and is estimated to be 8% dehydrated. Approximately what fluid volume should you give to rehydrate this dog?**
    A   500 ml
    B   1000 ml
    C   2000 ml
    D   2240 ml

2. **Which of the following solutions would you give intravenously to maintain an animal once it had been rehydrated?**
    A   Hartmann's solution
    B   Plasma
    C   5% dextrose
    D   0.18% sodium chloride, 4% dextrose (1/5 normal saline)

3. **If you wished to maintain a 36 kg dog on a drip, and you needed to give 2160 ml over 24 hours, how fast would you set the drip? (Assume that 1 ml = 20 drops)**
    A   1 drop per second
    B   1 drop every 2 seconds
    C   1 drop every 3 seconds
    D   2 drops per second

4. **Sodium bicarbonate should not be given with which of the following fluids?**
    A   Hartmann's solution
    B   Normal saline
    C   5% dextrose
    D   0.18% sodium chloride, 4% dextrose

5. **Over-infusion of a patient with intravenous fluids could lead to**
    A   The development of renal failure
    B   The development of oedema
    C   A fall in central venous pressure
    D   The development of hepatic failure

6. **The type of body water that makes up about 5% of an animal's total body weight is**
   A   Intracellular fluid
   B   Extracellular fluid
   C   Plasma
   D   Synovial fluid

7. **Which of the following conditions would result in a primary water deficit?**
   A   Unconsciousness
   B   Vomiting
   C   Diarrhoea
   D   Burns

8. **The anticoagulant used when collecting blood for blood transfusions is**
   A   Acid citrate dextrose (ACD)
   B   Heparin
   C   EDTA
   D   Fluoride oxalate

9. **Central venous pressure provides an indication of the state of an animal's circulation. What is normal central venous pressure in small animals?**
   A   3–7 cm H_2O
   B   150–160 mm H_2O
   C   3–7 mm Hg
   D   150–160 mm Hg

10. **All the following solutions are isotonic except**
    A   0.9% sodium chloride
    B   5% dextrose
    C   0.18% sodium chloride, 4% dextrose
    D   1.8% sodium chloride

11. **If an animal was suffering from chronic diarrhoea, which would be the most appropriate fluid to use for rehydration?**
    A   Normal saline
    B   5% dextrose
    C   Hartmann's solution
    D   0.18% sodium chloride, 4% dextrose

12. **A 4 kg cat normally has a PCV of 37%, but has become dehydrated and now has a PCV of 44%. How much fluid does it require for rehydration?**
    A   140 ml
    B   200 ml
    C   240 ml
    D   280 ml

13. **In which of the following cases might you need to supplement potassium in the drip?**
    A   An anorexic cat being maintained on intravenous fluids
    B   A pup with acute parvovirus infection
    C   A young adult dog that requires an enterotomy to remove a golf ball
    D   An older dog with a gastric torsion

14. **Concerning shock, which statement is the least accurate?**
    A   Shock is a maldistribution of blood flow, causing decreased delivery of oxygen to tissues
    B   Shock should be considered an emergency situation warranting immediate treatment
    C   Shock causes a marked parasympathetic response
    D   Shock can be caused by haemorrhage, severe stress, infection or anaphylaxis

The answers start on page 222

22 Anaesthesia and analgesia

32 Questions

1. **The premedicant agent that has significant analgesic effects is**
   A   Acepromazine
   B   Buprenorphine
   C   Atropine
   D   Diazepam

2. **The dose rate for buprenorphine is 0.006 mg/kg (6 µg/kg). The concentration of the solution is 0.3 mg/ml (300 µg/ml). How many ml does a 50 kg animal require?**
   A   0.1 ml
   B   0.5 ml
   C   1 ml
   D   2 ml

3. **Which problems are associated with the use of small animal Immobilon?**
   A   Hypotension and bradycardia
   B   Accidental self-administration
   C   Cyanosis due to hypoventilation
   D   All of the above

4. **The Magill circuit is classified as which type of breathing circuit?**
   A   Open
   B   Semi-open
   C   Semi-closed
   D   Closed

5. **Recovery from thiopentone-induced anaesthesia takes place through**
   A   Metabolism of the anaesthetic by the liver
   B   Redistribution of the thiopentone to fatty tissues, and then gradual metabolism by the liver
   C   Excretion of unchanged thiopentone by the kidney
   D   Exhalation of the anaesthetic

6. **All of the following anaesthetics can be used in the dog except**
   A Ketamine
   B Propofol
   C Alphaxalone and alphadolone acetate
   D Methohexitone sodium

7. **The Misuse of Drugs Act 1971 governs how the 'controlled drugs' must be stored and used. Which of the following falls into Schedule 3 of this Act?**
   A Diazepam
   B Butorphanol
   C Buprenorphine
   D Morphine

8. **Which of the following volatile anaesthetic agents must not be used with soda-lime?**
   A Isofluorane
   B Halothane
   C Ether
   D Trichloroethylene

9. **The pressure in a nitrous oxide cylinder decreases**
   A When the cylinder is half full
   B When all of the liquid nitrous oxide has vaporized, which occurs when the tank is nearly empty
   C If the cylinder is heated
   D As nitrous oxide is used from a full cylinder, thus providing an indication of the quantity of gas remaining

10. **Anticholinergics may be included in premedication for cats and dogs**
    A To produce pupil dilation
    B To decrease saliva and bronchial secretions
    C To decrease the amount of induction agent required
    D To calm the animal

11. **Which of the following is a narcotic?**
    A Pethidine
    B Xylazine
    C Ketamine
    D Propofol

12. Of the following drugs commonly used as premedicants, which does not cause a fall in blood pressure?
A   Xylazine (Rompun)
B   Acepromazine
C   Ketamine
D   Medetomidine (Domitor)

13. α_2-adrenoceptor agonists include the drugs xylazine and medetomidine. Which side-effect(s) may occur with their use in small animals?
A   Hypotension
B   Bradycardia
C   Respiratory depression
D   All of the above

14. What capacity is a size E oxygen cylinder?
A   680 litres
B   1360 litres
C   3400 litres
D   6800 litres

15. An analeptic is
A   A drug that causes drowsiness
B   A drug that produces calmness without drowsiness
C   A drug that stimulates the central nervous system
D   A drug that decreases the sensation of pain

16. Which of the following is a barbiturate anaesthetic?
A   Methohexitone sodium
B   Alphaxalone and alphadolone
C   Ketamine
D   Propofol

17. A neuro-leptanaesthetic is
A   A mixture of an opioid with an analgesic
B   A mixture of an analgesic with a premedicant
C   A mixture of a sedative with an inhalation anaesthetic
D   A mixture of a sedative with an opioid analgesic

18. **MAC numbers have been calculated for all the inhalation anaesthetics. Which of the following has the lowest MAC number?**
    A   Methoxyflurane
    B   Halothane
    C   Nitrous oxide
    D   Isoflurane

19. **Nitrous oxide and oxygen can be used together in anaesthesia. Which combination is usually used?**
    A   1 : 1 nitrous oxide : oxygen
    B   2 : 1 nitrous oxide : oxygen
    C   3 : 1 nitrous oxide : oxygen
    D   4 : 1 nitrous oxide : oxygen

20. **The anaesthetic used by Guedel to classify the stages of anaesthesia was**
    A   Chloroform
    B   Halothane
    C   Ether
    D   Thiopentone

21. **Different anaesthetic circuits require different fresh gas flow rates. Which circuit uses 1–1.5 × minute volume?**
    A   Lack
    B   Ayre's T-piece
    C   Bain
    D   Circle system

22. **Why are silicates included in soda-lime?**
    A   To keep the soda-lime dry
    B   To prevent the indicator dye from decomposing
    C   To prevent the soda-lime from forming an irritant dust
    D   To absorb the carbon dioxide

23. **Which of the following is a depolarizing neuromuscular blocker?**
    A   Neostigmine
    B   Suxamethonium
    C   Naloxone
    D   Vecuronium

24. **As an animal becomes anaesthetized, which is the first reflex to be lost?**
    A   Pedal reflex
    B   Anal reflex
    C   Swallowing reflex
    D   Palpebral reflex

25. **According to the Health and Safety Executive, what is the maximum length of tubing suitable for use with a passive scavenging system?**
    A   3 ft or 0.9 m
    B   5 ft or 1.5 m
    C   8.5 ft or 2.6 m
    D   12 ft or 3.7 m

26. **The anaesthetic gas supplied in blue cylinders is**
    A   Oxygen
    B   Nitrous oxide
    C   Carbon dioxide
    D   Cyclopropane

27. **Activated charcoal within a circuit removes which of the following?**
    A   Carbon dioxide
    B   Halothane
    C   Nitrous oxide
    D   Halothane and nitrous oxide

28. **The dose rate for thiopentone is 10 mg/kg, and you have been given a 2.5% solution. How many ml would you need to draw up for a 50 g mouse?**
    A   0.2 ml
    B   0.02 ml
    C   0.5 ml
    D   5 ml

29. **The intravenous anaesthetic with the shortest recovery time is**
    A   Propofol
    B   Thiopentone
    C   Methohexitone
    D   Ketamine with diazepam

30. **Under Guedel's classification, which stage**
    of anaesthesia is surgical anaesthesia?
    A   Stage I
    B   Stage II
    C   Stage III
    D   Stage IV

31. **Muscle relaxants act at which site within the nervous system?**
    A   The neuromuscular junction
    B   The nerve axon
    C   The brain
    D   The spinal cord

32. **Calculate the fresh gas flow rate needed for a 4 kg cat**
    using an Ayre's T-piece with Jackson Rees modification.
    Which of the following would be suitable to use?
    A   300 ml/min
    B   800 ml/min
    C   1000 ml/min
    D   2000 ml/min

The answers start on page   *226*

23 Radiography

24 Questions

1. **The grid factor for a grid depends on which of the following?**
   A   Grid ratio
   B   The number of lines per centimetre
   C   The thickness of the lines
   D   All of the above

2. **A veterinary surgeon has performed a contrast study of the urethra by introducing contrast medium via a urinary catheter. Which of the following terms would describe this technique?**
   A   Intravenous urography
   B   Ureterography
   C   Positive contrast cystography
   D   Retrograde urethrography

3. **A 20 kg dog's metacarpal is radiographed using the following exposure factors: FFD = 70 cm, kV = 45 kV, mA = 20 mA, time = 0.3 secs. What are the new exposure factors if the time is increased to 0.4 secs?**
   A   FFD = 70 cm, kV = 40 kV, mA = 20 mA
   B   FFD = 70 cm, kV = 45 kV, mA = 15 mA
   C   FFD = 75 cm, kV = 45 kV, mA = 20 mA
   D   FFD = 70 cm, kV = 45 kV, mA = 27 mA

4. **In which part of the X-ray film are the radiation-sensitive grains found?**
   A   Supercoat
   B   Subbing layer
   C   Emulsion
   D   Base

5. **Altering which exposure factor will affect the quality of the X-ray beam produced?**
   A   mA
   B   Time
   C   Focal-film distance
   D   kV

6. **The absorption of X-rays by a tissue depends on which of the following?**
   A   Its atomic number
   B   The density of the tissue
   C   The thickness of the tissue
   D   All of the above

7. **The processing sequence for a radiograph is development, fixing and washing. What takes place in the fixer?**
   A   Exposed silver grains are washed off the film
   B   Unexposed silver bromide grains are reduced to metallic silver
   C   Exposed silver bromide grains are reduced to metallic silver
   D   Unexposed silver bromide grains are washed off the film

8. **Which type of contrast medium would be suitable for use in a myelogram?**
   A   High osmolar, ionic water-soluble iodine preparation
   B   Barium compound
   C   Low osmolar, non-ionic water-soluble iodine preparation
   D   Any of the above

9. **The greatest amount of radiation a person may legally receive in a year is the**
   A   Recommended safety dose
   B   Minimum permissible dose
   C   Maximum permissible dose
   D   Maximum mAs

10. **The use of X-rays in practice is controlled by which piece of legislation?**
    A   Health and Safety at Work Act
    B   COSHH Regulations
    C   Guidance Notes for the Protection of Persons against Ionising Radiations arising from Veterinary Use
    D   Ionising Radiations Regulations 1999

11. **If you examined a radiograph that had been overexposed, how would it appear?**
    A   'Soot and whitewash' film – white subject, dark background, with no internal detail visible
    B   Black background, subject detail too dark – a flat film lacking contrast
    C   Subject pale, background grey and fails the 'finger test'
    D   One area of the radiograph black – generally unrelated to the position of the primary beam

12. **If the distance between the effective focal spot and the object being radiographed is trebled, by how much should you increase the exposure factors to maintain the same radiographic density?**
    A   Increase mAs by three times
    B   Increase kV by three times
    C   Increase mAs by nine times
    D   Increase kV by nine times

13. **All of the following are properties of X-rays except**
    A   They travel in straight lines
    B   They affect photographic emulsion
    C   They can penetrate all materials to some degree
    D   They can be reflected by some materials

14. **Which statement is true about different types of grid?**
    A   Potter Bucky is a stationary grid
    B   Parallel grids can result in grid cut-off at the edge of the radiograph
    C   Focused and pseudo-focused grids are the same type of grid
    D   For all types of grid, the exposure factors needed are lower than without the grid

15. **Heat is lost in the rotating anode X-ray tube head by**
    A   Conduction through copper
    B   Convection through air
    C   Radiation through the vacuum
    D   Evaporation

16. **There is a step-up transformer within the X-ray tube head. Why is this needed?**
    A   To change alternating current into direct current
    B   To reduce the voltage to the filament from 240 V to 10 V
    C   To increase the voltage between the anode and cathode from 240 V to 40–80 kV
    D   To prevent fluctuations in the voltage from the mains

17. **If you were developing non-screen film manually, how much longer would you leave the film in the developer compared with screen film?**
    A   Double the normal developing time
    B   Increase by 2 minutes
    C   Increase by 1 minute
    D   Increase by 30 seconds

18. **A dog is radiographed using the following exposure factors:**
kV = 70 kV, mA = 20 mA, time = 0.2 secs, FFD = 70 cm.
You want to introduce a grid with grid factor 4.
Which of the following settings could you use?
A   kV = 70 kV, mA = 40 mA, time = 0.2 secs, FFD = 70 cm
B   kV = 80 kV, mA = 20 mA, time = 0.2 secs, FFD = 70 cm
C   kV = 80 kV, mA = 40 mA, time = 0.2 secs, FFD = 70 cm
D   kV = 70 kV, mA = 40 mA, time = 0.4 secs, FFD = 80 cm

19. **The radius of the controlled area from the X-ray**
tube head when used in an unconfined area is
A   1 m
B   2 m
C   3 m
D   4 m

20. **Which of the following newer imaging techniques also**
uses an X-ray tube head to generate its images?
A   Computed tomography (CT scanning)
B   Magnetic resonance imaging
C   Ultrasound
D   Scintigraphy

21. **The production of scattered radiation can be reduced**
by doing all of the following except
A   Compressing the part being radiographed
B   Collimating the beam
C   Using a grid
D   Using a lead-backed cassette

22. **The statement about screens that is incorrect is**
A   Radiation causes crystals in the screens to fluoresce
B   Screens mean that higher exposure factors are required
C   Screens reduce the definition of the radiograph
D   Screen crystals can be made of calcium tungstate

23. There is an aluminium filter incorporated into the window of the X-ray tube head. What is its function?
  A   To absorb X-ray beams leaving the tube head at the wrong angle
  B   To absorb any low energy X-rays
  C   To prevent light getting into the X-ray tube head
  D   To absorb heat

24. Developer solutions should be kept in a tank with the lid on
  A   To prevent evaporation
  B   To prevent contamination with dust
  C   To prevent oxidation of the developer chemicals
  D   To prevent inhalation of the developer chemicals during times other than processing

The answer start on page   *235*

Answers

1 Handling, control, observation and care of the patient

1. D *A dark green vulval discharge in a bitch due to whelp without any signs of straining would give cause for concern*
A dark green vulval discharge would indicate that the placentae were starting to separate from the uterine wall. This is normally seen when the bitch gives birth, but if the bitch was not straining the pups would rapidly die without an oxygen supply. It is likely that a Caesarean section would need to be performed to try to save the pups.
Pink mucous membranes and a capillary refill time of 1–2 seconds are both normal signs of a healthy circulation.
Tom cats often pass a slightly cloudy urine due to the presence of mucus and some crystals.

2. C *An animal in pain may show tachypnoea*
Hypothermia is an abnormally low body temperature. Animals in pain usually have an elevated temperature. Icterus means jaundice or yellow discoloration of the mucous membranes and sclera. This indicates either liver disease, increased red blood cell breakdown or an obstruction to bile flow.
Bradycardia is an abnormally slow heart rate. Animals in pain generally have a rapid heart rate described as a tachycardia.

3. C *Tenesmus means straining*
Haematuria means blood in the urine, dyschezia is difficulty passing faeces and epiphora describes the overflow of tears.

4. C *Fatty faeces can be described as steatorrhoea*
Diarrhoea simply means that the faeces are more fluid than normal. Dyschezia and faecal tenesmus both mean difficulty in passing faeces, or straining to pass faeces.

5. B *Blepharospasm means screwing up the eyelids*
A dislike of bright light is photophobia.
Excessive tear production is epiphora.
Oedematous conjunctiva is chemosis.

6. C *Epistaxis means bleeding from the nose*

7. A *The normal temperature for a cat is 38.0–38.5°C (100.4–101.6°F)*

8. C *Haemoptysis means coughing up blood*
Vomiting blood is referred to as haematemesis. Blood in the anterior chamber of the eye is hyphaema, and blood in faeces is described as melaena.

9. B *After reduction of a dislocated hip an Ehmer sling can be applied*
The Ehmer sling, also called the figure-of-eight bandage, keeps the hindlimb in a flexed position and prevents the animal from weight bearing on that leg. This is usually left on for a few days until the soft tissue reaction subsides.
    Esmarch's bandage is a rubber bandage used as a tourniquet. It is most commonly used for surgery on distal limbs, such as the amputation of a digit, when it is helpful to have a bloodless operating field.
    The Robert–Jones bandage is a bulky support bandage used sometimes in first aid to support limb fractures, or applied after surgery to provide comfort and support for a limb.
    The Velpeau sling is applied to the forelimb to prevent weight-bearing, and can be used after shoulder surgery.

10. B *Tape muzzles could be used quite easily in all types of dog except brachycephalic breeds*
Brachycephalic breeds, such as the Pug or Pekingese, have very foreshortened nasal chambers, and so there is little nose to take any type of muzzle.
    Doliocephalic animals have very long nasal chambers, and include breeds such as the Rough Collie or some of the hounds, for example the Borzoi.
    Mesaticephalic or mesocephalic animals have average length nasal chambers. Breeds include Labradors, Cocker spaniels and most of the terriers.

11. B *The vein most commonly used to administer intravenous injections in the dog is the cephalic vein*
It is, however, possible to use any of the veins listed. The jugular vein is useful for the administration of intravenous fluids in collapsed patients. The sublingual vein is often used during anaesthesia, when access to other superficial veins in the body may be limited because of the sterile surgical field. The saphenous vein tends to be used when there is a problem with the use of the cephalic veins.

12. C *The maximum volume of drug that should be given by intramuscular injection in the dog is 5 ml*

13. C *It would be best to keep a hospital ward at a temperature of 18°C*

It is important that hospitalized patients are kept warm. Hypothermia or lowering of core body temperature will at least delay recovery, and in many cases will allow the animal's condition to become worse.

14. D *Local heat can be used in the treatment of abscesses*

Heat causes vasodilation, and so increases the blood supply to a particular area. This can be helpful in bringing white cells to an area of infection. It also draws abscesses to a head, such that they can then be lanced and drained.

Cold applications can be used in the management of the other conditions listed.

2 First aid

1. **A** *Haemorrhage from the distal tail can be controlled by occluding the coccygeal artery*
The coccygeal artery runs along the ventral surface of the vertebrae of the tail, and it can be pressed against the bones sufficiently to control the bleeding.

   The femoral artery and the brachial artery can also be compressed against bone in the same way to control bleeding in the hind and fore limbs respectively. The aorta lies within the thorax and abdomen and is therefore not accessible.

2. **C** *Blepharospasm could be caused by ocular trauma*
Blepharospasm means screwing up the eyelids.

3. **D** *An aural haematoma is an example of a closed wound*
A closed wound is one in which the surface of the skin or mucous membrane has not been breached, although there is damage to the tissues beneath.

   A wound in which skin or mucous membrane is damaged is referred to as an open wound.

4. **A** *The cat with pale clammy mucous membranes, fast shallow respiration and subnormal temperature is the animal with the most seriously life-threatening condition and should therefore be seen first*
Remember, the order for emergency treatment is to check airway, breathing, circulation, haemorrhage and shock. Problems in any of these areas can be fatal, and the signs given for the cat in this question are those of severe shock.

   The dog, although it has a fractured femur, is less severely shocked and fractures rarely cause death, so this can wait until the cat has been looked after.

   Bee stings may lead to severe problems, but this is usually when they occur in the mouth or pharynx, when the swelling might be sufficient to occlude the airway. The other situation in which they are a serious problem is if an animal suffers an anaphylactic reaction to the sting. Respiratory problems would become apparent very quickly in this case.

5. **C** *The term used to describe a fracture in which the fragments have damaged other vital structures is complicated fracture*
Compound fractures are open fractures in which there is a wound overlying the fracture, so that the fracture is open to the environment.

A comminuted fracture is when the bone is broken in one place, but there are several fragments.

A multiple fracture is when a bone is broken in more than one site, or more than one bone is fractured.

6. D *Splinting would be appropriate for midshaft radius and ulna fractures*
Splints can only be applied to fractures distal to the elbow and stifle, since for a splint to be effective it must immobilize the joints above and below the fracture site.

7. B *A sprain is an injury to a ligament within a joint caused by excess stress*
A strain is an injury to a muscle or tendon caused by overstretching.

8. C *A tourniquet should never be left in place longer than 15 minutes*
If the haemorrhage has not been controlled in this time, the tourniquet should be loosened slowly, blood allowed to circulate freely for at least a minute, and the tourniquet then reapplied. Tourniquets should only be used as a last resort for haemorrhage control.

9. A *The pup that had chewed through an electric cable and was unconscious should be treated first*
The first thing to do is to make the area safe by turning off the power to the cable. It is important that you check the animal has an airway, is breathing and its circulation is functioning adequately before attending to the other patients.

10. C *Cardiac compression should be applied 80 times per minute for a large dog.*
The aim in cardiac massage is to mimic the natural heart rate of the animal. For a small dog or cat a faster rate would be needed, up to 120 compressions per minute.

11. B *Reactionary or intermediate haemorrhage is seen 24–48 hours after the incident while the vessel wall is undergoing repair*
Haemorrhage can start again at this time as blood pressure increases and returns to normal. This may be sufficient to displace the clot that had formed.

Haemorrhage seen at the time of injury is primary haemorrhage.

A haemorrhage seen 3–10 days afterward injury is usually due to infection or necrosis of the vessel and is called secondary haemorrhage.

12. A *The client should be advised to keep the tissues moist and to bring the hamster down to the surgery*
The most likely problem in this case is a rectal prolapse, which is fairly common in hamsters. If it has only just occurred the tissue may not be too traumatized and swollen, and it may be returned quite easily. However, prolapses often recur and a purse-string suture may be needed. If the tissue has been out for any time it may have become devitalized and damaged, in which case surgery will be necessary.

13. A *An animal with a prolapsed eyeball should always be seen immediately*
If this condition is treated quickly, the eye can be replaced and saved. If it is left, the eye rapidly becomes dried out and the optic nerve becomes stretched and can be permanently damaged so that the animal loses its sight from that eye.

The other conditions listed can all be serious in some instances, but also may not *have* to be seen immediately. You should question the owner carefully to obtain a full and accurate history so that you have an indication of the severity of the condition.

14. C *The Heimlich manoeuvre is used for dislodging a pharyngeal foreign body*
A foreign body in the pharynx can cause an airway obstruction, and if it cannot be removed easily, then the Heimlich manoeuvre should be tried.

15. D *The Veterinary Surgeons Act 1966 states that lay persons may administer first aid in an emergency*

16. C *The thing that should be done immediately after checking its airway and breathing is to keep the dog warm*
The dog is in shock, and it is very important that the animal's body temperature is not allowed to fall too far below normal. The veterinary surgeon should be called after covering the animal with something to keep it warm.

17. B *The first thing that should be done for an animal suffering from heat stroke is to cool it with cold water*
The water evaporating from the skin will produce quite rapid cooling of the body. It is important to monitor the animal's body temperature while doing this, as the temperature should not be allowed to fall too rapidly, or to drop below normal.

18. D *A reducible hernia describes the situation in which abdominal contents have passed through a natural hole in the body wall, but can be pushed back through this*
A rupture is similar, except that the abdominal contents have passed through a tear in the body wall rather than through a natural opening.

19. B *In wound healing, monocytes and macrophages clear cellular debris*
Monocytes and macrophages are phagocytes, and they engulf and digest dead and dying tissue from wounds. Monocytes and macrophages are very similar to each other the difference being that monocytes circulate in the blood while macrophages are found within tissues.
New capillaries develop within the wound, which bring nutrients to the site, and fibroblasts lay down collagen. Together these form granulation tissue. Fibroblasts also assist in wound contraction.

20. C *You should not attempt to reduce the dislocation*
It is important that the dislocation is not considered in isolation, and the whole animal should be checked for other problems, particularly for any affecting the airway, breathing or circulation. The animal should be encouraged to rest and treated for shock.

21. D *An animal in shock should not be given food and water*
Oxygen and intravenous fluids will be helpful in all types of shock, and in most cases antibiotics are given as protection against potential secondary infections developing.

22. B *Deep unconsciousness could be distinguished from death by checking the colour of the mucous membranes*
In both deep unconsciousness and death the pupils would be widely dilated, there would be no pedal reflexes, and the animal's muscles would be flaccid. However the mucous membranes would be quite different in colour – pale or slightly blue in a deeply unconscious animal, but ashen grey in a dead animal.

23. D *Subcutaneous emphysema is air under the skin*

24. C *Nystagmus can develop after a 'stroke-like' event*
Nystagmus is the involuntary flicking of the eyes in one
direction. It usually occurs in association with damage to the
vestibular system within the inner ear, or central nervous
system lesions such as 'strokes' or tumours affecting the brain.
Strictly speaking, animals do not have the same type of strokes
as humans; however, they suffer from conditions that generate
similar clinical signs, so these are usually referred to as strokes.

25. C *Increased body temperature is not usually seen in shock*
In most cases the animal will have a subnormal temperature.
Pale mucous membranes, tachycardia and a weak pulse are
common findings in shock.

3 Poisons

1. C *The specific antidote that can be given to an animal suspected of having been poisoned with organophosphates is atropine sulphate*
Sodium calcium edetate in saline solution is used specifically for lead poisoning. Ethanol and sodium bicarbonate are used in the management of ingestion of ethylene glycol, and acetyl cysteine can be given after paracetamol poisoning.

2. C *Animals with ethylene glycol poisoning often develop calcium oxalate crystals within their urine*

3. B *Paraquat poisoning causes severe renal damage and respiratory distress*
The animal will usually die due to a severe interstitial pneumonia, which leads to progressive respiratory failure. Chronic lead poisoning produces nervous signs such as disorientation, ataxia and blindness.
Changes in coat pigmentation are not usually seen in small animal poisoning cases.

4. D *The pesticide with an anaesthetic action that causes a dramatic drop in body temperature and leads to hypothermia and death is alphachloralose*
This is found in some rodenticides.
Sodium chlorate affects haemoglobin within the blood, and causes depression, anorexia, abdominal pain and haematuria.
Paraquat is a very potent poison, leading to depression, vomiting, diarrhoea, progressive dyspnoea and death within 10 days.
Metaldehyde produces neurological signs, including incoordination, loss of consciousness, convulsions and cyanosis.

5. D *Acetyl cysteine can be used in the management of animals suspected of having been poisoned by paracetamol*

6. D *Vomiting should not be induced if poisoning by bleach, phenol or petroleum products is suspected*
Vomiting should not be induced in any patient that is unconscious, convulsing or that has ingested an irritant or volatile poison. Bleach and phenol are both very irritant, and petroleum products are volatile.

7. C *Warfarin is used legally as a rodenticide*

8. D *Carbon monoxide, sodium chlorate and paracetamol all produce changes in haemoglobin, which lead to a colour change of the blood*
Sodium chlorate and paracetamol both change haemoglobin into methaemoglobin. This results in the mucous membranes appearing a muddy brown colour.

Carbon monoxide is carried by haemoglobin in preference to oxygen, and instead of the blood appearing a dark red colour it lightens to a cherry-red colour. This can be misleading because, without looking carefully, the animal can appear to have a healthy colour, suggesting that normal oxygenation of tissues is occurring. In fact the tissues are hypoxic, as carbon monoxide cannot be used by them and there is little oxygen available.

4 Occupational hazards and human first aid

1. C *Special waste refers to bottles and vials that have been contaminated with drug products and which should be stored in yellow plastic bins until collected and incinerated by an authorized collector*
Waste contaminated with animal tissues, blood or excretions is clinical waste. This should be stored in yellow sacks, and collected and incinerated by an authorized collector. Animal bodies are also a type of clinical waste, although owners may bury their own animals at home. Other non-hazardous waste generated by a veterinary practice is industrial waste, which can be collected as normal refuse by the local council or other collector.
The legislation covering this area of practice is The Environmental Protection Act 1990.

2. D *The piece of legislation described is the Control of Substances Hazardous to Health (COSHH) Regulations 1988*
These Regulations form part of a series of Regulations that fit within the framework of the Health and Safety At Work Act 1974. The series also includes the Health and Safety (First Aid) Regulations 1981, which cover the level of first aid expertise and equipment a business should have, and RIDDOR, which dictates that any incident where someone is badly injured at work, or falls ill through a major infectious disease, must be reported to the Health and Safety Executive. The Controlled Waste Regulations 1992 is one of three pieces of legislation that cover business' responsibilities to the environment.

3. A *The elevated sling can be used in the support of a fractured collar bone*
The arm sling should be used in the other examples given.

4. B *Tourniquets should NEVER be used in human first aid*
All the other actions are appropriate management for a severe bleed from a limb.

5. C *In these circumstances, the first action to take is to call an ambulance*
The most likely reason for an adult to collapse with no obvious case is a heart attack, and research has shown that the victim's chances of survival depend largely on the speed with

which they get professional help. Therefore the current recommendation is to assume that the person has suffered a heart attack and call the ambulance accordingly. Once this is done the patient should be reassessed, and then cardiac and respiratory resuscitation can be started.

6. D *In human first aid, the sequence for cardio-pulmonary resuscitation of an adult is two breaths and 15 compressions* This needs to be given at a rate such that 100 cardiac compressions are completed within a minute. This allows for the fact that cardiac massage is only about 70% successful, and not every compression squeezes the heart effectively.

7. C *The Accident Book should be kept for a minimum of 3 years after the last entry*

8. A *The most appropriate treatment would be to get the person to lie down and raise and support the legs* Without knowing the reason for the shock it is not advisable to give oral fluids, although a little water may be used just to moisten the patient's lips. Someone in shock should never be disregarded; just as in animals, this can be a life-threatening condition, and the patient should never be left alone for any time.

9. D *All of the burns described will need further medical attention* Only small superficial burns can be considered as minor, and these should be cooled with cold water for at least 10 minutes, jewellery or other constricting items removed, and the area then dressed. If there is any doubt as to the severity of the burn, further medical advice should be sought.

10. C *The RICE mnemonic is used as an aid to remembering the treatment for sprains*
R = Rest,
I = Ice,
C = Compress,
E = Elevate.
Therefore, the sprained joint should be rested, cooled with ice packs, bandaged firmly and elevated.

5 Management of kennels and catteries

1. A *The quarantine period in the United Kingdom is 6 months*

2. A *The bitch due to be speyed should be cleaned out first*
It is important if one nurse is involved cleaning out inpatients in a hospital kennel that attempts are made to minimize the risk of spread of infection. Animals with infectious diseases should be left until last, so that the pathogens are not carried to other animals. Ideally, these animals should be looked after by a different person from the nurse caring for the uninfected animals.

3. B *The minimum temperature at which a kennel or cattery should be kept is 7°C*
This is the minimum temperature recommended in the *BVA Guide to District Authorities and their Veterinary Inspectors*. However, this is only suitable for fit and healthy animals. Hospitalized patients or breeding animals require a warmer environmental temperature.

4. C *The minimum height of a dog kennel in a quarantine kennel is 1.8 m*

5. B *The Bichon Frise is a member of the Toy Group*
The whippet is a hound, the Lhasa Apso is a member of the utility group, and the Dandie Dinmont is a terrier.

6. C *At least six air changes per hour should take place in a kennel block to minimize the risk of respiratory infections*

7. A *The hypochlorites are unsuitable for skin usage*
The hypochlorites or bleaches are extremely irritant to skin, and care should be taken when they are used that they do not come into direct contact with any animals.
     They are, however, cheap and very effective environmental disinfectants. They are active against almost all fungi, bacteria and viruses, and can be used in food areas.

8. B *Chlorhexidine is an example of a diguanide*
Formaldehyde is an aldehyde, povidone-iodine is an iodophor, one of the halogen disinfectants, and cetrimide is a quaternary ammonium compound.

9. C *Records of quarantined animals should be kept for at least 1 year after their release from quarantine*

10. C *The cat that is long-haired is the Ragdoll*

11. B *After arrival in the UK, an owner has to wait 2 weeks before being allowed to visit his or her own animal in quarantine*
It is possible to visit the animal earlier than this if special authorization is granted.

12. C *Glutaraldehyde is unsafe to use on skin*
Glutaraldehyde is extremely irritant to skin, and also to the respiratory tract.
   Chlorhexidine, cetrimide and povidone-iodine can all be used on skin at low concentrations, but at higher concentrations these too can be tissue-toxic.

13. D *Friar's balsam, silver nitrate and ferric chloride can all be used as styptics*

14. A *Disinfection is defined as the destruction of micro-organisms but not necessarily bacterial spores*
Sterilization is the destruction of micro-organisms including bacterial spores, and antisepsis is the removal of micro-organisms but not necessarily bacterial spores on skin or living tissues. This can also be called skin disinfection.

15. A *The Basenji is a hound*

16. C *Animals in boarding kennels should be checked at least every 4 hours during the day*
This is the recommendation made in the *BVA Guide to District Authorities and their Veterinary Inspectors.*

17. C *Contaminated sharps should be placed in rigid plastic containers and then incinerated*
The opening to the plastic containers should be too small for someone to get a hand into, and the containers should be collected by an authorized collecting company and then incinerated. These containers should be yellow, like the clinical waste bags.

18. D *The design of a quarantine kennel must incorporate the provision of observation panels, traps and solid partitions between kennels*
This is specified in the Rabies Order 1974, which gives details for the construction of quarantine kennels.

19. C *Phenols are particularly toxic to cats*
Phenol disinfectants are irritant to all species but they are particularly toxic to cats, and produce signs of vomiting, diarrhoea and abdominal pain and, in severe cases, convulsions, coma and death.

22. B *The Birman has white socks on all four feet*

21. A *Quaternary ammonium compounds have mild detergent properties and inactivate phenol and hypochlorite disinfectants*

22. C *The legislation that provides detailed information about the necessary design and construction of a quarantine kennel is The Rabies Order 1974*
The Animal Boarding Establishment Act 1963 gives general guidelines for any boarding facility.

Before any kennel or cattery can be built planning permission must be granted, as stated in the Town and Country Planning Act 1971.

The Breeding of Dogs Act 1973 requires that any person owning two or more bitches and breeding for profit must be licensed by the district council.

23. D *In order to travel under the Pets Travel Scheme, all statements must be complied with*
This Scheme allows dogs and cats to travel between certain countries and the UK providing that they meet particular criteria. As stated in the question, they must be microchipped, vaccinated and blood tested. This must take place at least 6 months before their entry into the UK. Only certain ports and airports will be used as entry points, and all animals must be treated for ticks and tapeworm before leaving the continent. Animals failing to meet these requirements will still have to undergo quarantine, as will animals being imported from countries not included in the scheme.

6 Practice organization, management, law and ethics

1. C *A trainee veterinary nurse may descale and polish teeth at the direction of his/her employer*
Under Schedule 3 of the Veterinary Surgeons Act 1966, only a *qualified* veterinary nurse whose name appears on the Register of Veterinary Nurses may perform minor surgery that does not involve entering a body cavity. This would include suturing wounds.

A trainee veterinary nurse or other lay staff may undertake some procedures such as suture removal, descaling and polishing teeth, changing dressings and trimming claws and beaks. These are not considered to be surgical procedures.

Under current legislation, no one other than a veterinary surgeon may perform castrations on companion animals because this involves entry into the abdominal cavity (by virtue of cutting the tunica vaginalis).

2. D *All the statements are requirements of the Dangerous Dogs Act 1991*
The breeds affected by the Dangerous Dogs Act are American Pit Bull terriers, Japanese Tosas, Dogo Argentinos and Fila Brazilieros. The requirements of tattooing, neutering, identichipping and registering had to be completed by November 1991, and any dogs of these breeds found to be in violation of the law after this date are to be or have already been euthanased.

3. B *If a client comes to the surgery asking for a second opinion, the original veterinary surgeon should be informed*
This is a matter of ethics, and is to avoid unscrupulous veterinary surgeons taking another surgeon's clients without his or her knowledge.

4. D *The RCVS recommends that client records should be kept for 6 years after an animal has died or the owners have moved away*

5. D *'Dead files' is the term used to describe information that has been kept longer than is actually necessary*

6. B *Supersession arises when a veterinary surgeon takes over a client from another veterinary surgeon without the latter's knowledge*

7. D *The Veterinary Surgeons Act 1966 provides details about the practice of veterinary medicine and surgery in the United Kingdom*
The Protection of Animals Acts 1911–1988 set out what constitutes cruelty to animals, and define the actions that are punishable by fines or imprisonment.

The Protection of Animals (Anaesthetics) Acts 1954 and 1964 are part of these acts, but specifically deal with procedures that should be carried out with the use of anaesthetics, and list which procedures are exempt from this requirement.

The Medicines Act 1968 governs the classification, manufacture, importation and dispensing of all medicinal products. This includes drugs used in human medicine as well as veterinary medicine.

8. D *All the statements are offences under UK law*
All animals used for scientific procedures must be bred by licensed establishments. Stray or stolen pets are never allowed to be used, under The Animals (Scientific Procedures) Act 1986. Organizing or advertising fights between animals is outlawed by The Protection of Animals (Amendment) Act 1988. The Protection of Animals Acts also make it illegal for someone to cause suffering to an animal through failing to do something – whether or not the cruelty was intentional.

9. C *The Breeding of Dogs Act 1973 requires a property to be licensed if there are two or more bitches used for breeding and the pups are to be sold for profit*

7 Nutrition

1. **B** *In cats, a deficiency in taurine can cause retinal degeneration*
   Most species can synthesize taurine from other amino acids, but cats are unable to do this. Lack of taurine in the diet leads to retinal degeneration, decreased fertility and failure of bile salts production so that fats cannot be digested normally.

   Deficiencies in Vitamin A lead to corneal ulceration, conjunctivitis, ataxia and skin lesions.

   Methionine and tryptophan are both essential amino acids and are needed for normal growth and development.

2. **D** *The vitamin that affects the growth and mineralization of bones and increases calcium absorption from the intestine is Vitamin D*
   Vitamin A is also involved with normal development of bones and teeth, but does not affect calcium uptake from the intestine.

   Thiamine and nicotinic acid are both members of the B group vitamins, and are needed as co-enzymes for metabolic reactions in the body.

3. **B** *The basal metabolic rate is the amount of energy a healthy animal doing nothing uses in a day*

4. **C** *Guinea pigs cannot synthesize Vitamin C, so must have an adequate supply within their diet*
   Vitamins A, B and D are essential in the diets of all animals.

5. **C** *A diet consisting solely of lean meat would be deficient in calcium, phosphorus and the fat-soluble vitamins*

6. **A** *Yeast is a good source of B vitamins*

7. **D** *Growing animals should be fed a diet containing calcium and phosphorus in the ratio 1 : 1*
   Imbalances in dietary calcium and phosphorus manifest as skeletal abnormalities such as growth plate deformities. Owners should therefore be dissuaded from over-supplementing calcium in the diet.

8. **A** *Excess vitamin A in the diet could result in excessive bone proliferation, leading to the eventual fusion of vertebrae and limb bones*
   This is seen most frequently in cats that have been fed diets consisting mainly of liver. Many bones are affected, especially the vertebrae and limb bones. The condition is quite painful

while the new bone is being deposited, and results in restriction of movement for the animal.

Vitamin E deficiency results in steatitis (inflammation of fat), muscle dystrophies and gestation failure. Lack of vitamin B is unusual, as many B vitamins are synthesized by bacteria within the intestines. Vitamin K is not very toxic in excess, but may cause anaemias in young animals.

9. C *Copper is needed within the body for haemoglobin synthesis*
Copper is also needed for melanin synthesis.

The thyroid hormones contain iodine, which is why it is required as a trace element within the diet. Calcium, phosphorus and magnesium are needed for bone production, and sodium, potassium and calcium are all needed for normal nerve and muscle function.

10. A *Increasing fibre in the diet can be beneficial for animals with colitis*
There are several diseases that can improve if dietary fibre is increased, and together these are referred to as 'fibre-responsive diseases'. These include colitis, diabetes mellitus and obesity.

For the management of pancreatitis and acute enteritis, the aim is to provide a very light, highly digestible diet which is low in fat and contains simple nutrients.

Sodium should be restricted in the diet of patients with cardiac disease so that water is not retained by the body and the workload of the heart is decreased.

11. C *A diet low in protein, high in B vitamins and with increased carbohydrate is required for animals suffering from renal disease*
The type of diet for animals with renal disease contains low quantities of high-quality protein to try and minimize the production of urea, which has to be cleared by the kidneys. The carbohydrates are increased to replace the calories that would normally be generated by the protein, and B vitamins are increased to replace those that are lost in the urine due to the polyuria.

Obese animals and those with diabetes mellitus require high fibre diets, and in both of these conditions the precise quantities of food eaten should be regulated carefully.

Animals with malabsorption syndromes require foods that are highly digestible and contain nutrients of high biological value so that their nutritional needs can be met from a relatively small amount of food.

12. **D** *Thiamin and pantothenic acid are both B vitamins*
Tryptophan is an amino acid, and ascorbic acid is more commonly known as vitamin C.

8 Genetics

1. D *Epistasis is the term used to describe the phenotypic effect of one gene obscuring the effect of another gene*
Errors produced in DNA result in mutations.
    Two genes on the same chromosomes that are often inherited together are said to be linked or to show linkage.
    Alternative forms of a gene at the same gene locus are called alleles.

2. C *A sex-limited gene is found on the autosomal chromosomes, but only expressed in animals of one sex*
Sex-linked genes are found on the sex chromosomes, that is the X and Y chromosomes.

3. A *The name given to the position of a gene on a chromosome is the gene locus*
Alleles are alternative forms of genes at the same gene locus.
    The centromere is the region of a chromosome that is drawn towards the centriole during mitosis and meiosis.
    Autosome is the word used to describe any chromosome except the sex chromosomes.

4. B *The characteristic that is true of mitosis but not of meiosis is that the daughter cells are identical to each other*
    In mitosis, two daughter cells are produced that are identical to each other and to the parent cell. Most cells of the body divide in this way.
    In meiosis, two consecutive divisions take place such that four daughter cells are produced. These are not the same as each other or the parent cell, and they only contain half the genetic information of the parent cell, having just one copy of each chromosome. Only the sex cells divide this way to produce the sperm and ova.

5. A *An animal that has two identical alleles for a particular gene is described as being homozygous*
A heterozygous animal has two different alleles for a gene, and a hemizygous animal only has one allele for a particular gene. The main instance in which this arises is in the male animal, which only has one copy of genes on the non-pairing section of the X chromosome. Homologous is the word used to describe the chromosomes that pair up together in the nucleus and have the same gene loci along their length.

6. A *Mendel's Second Law states that each pair of genes separates independently from others*
This was perfectly true for the characteristics that Mendel was studying. However, due to the structure of chromosomes there is a strong likelihood that genes that sit adjacent to each other will be inherited together. This phenomenon is known as linkage.
The other three statements all form part of Mendel's First Law.

7. B *If two blue Dobermans were mated, all the pups would be blue*
To be blue-coated, both the parents can only have genes for blue coat colouring. Therefore this is the only gene that each parent can pass to the pups, so the pups must also be blue.

8. B *The defect that is inherited but not congenital is progressive retinal atrophy*
Inherited defects are controlled through the genes an animal inherits from its parents. They may or may not be present at birth. Congenital defects are defects that are present at birth regardless of their cause.
Progressive retinal atrophy is inherited, but does not develop in affected animals until they are several years old.
Umbilical hernias, Collie eye anomaly and cleft palate can be inherited, but are all present from birth.

9. C *If a bitch is mated to a dog to whom she is related, though not closely, this is described as line breeding*
Inbreeding describes when very close relatives are mated – for example sibling matings, or daughter to sire matings.
Outbreeding is when animals are mated which are less closely related than if selected at random.

10. C *To determine whether a black cat is carrying the tabby gene, it should be mated to a tabby cat*
This is an example of 'backcross to the recessive'. If any of the offspring are tabby, then the black cat must have been carrying the tabby gene.
If all the offspring are black, then it is likely that the black cat did not carry the tabby gene.

11. B *If two genes are said to be linked, they are often inherited together*

Linked genes are often inherited together because they lie on the same chromosome and are close enough not to be separated by the crossover events that can occur during meiosis.

The nearer the two gene loci are to each other, the more likely they are to be inherited together, and the linkage is described as being close.

12. A *The term genotype is used to describe the genetic make-up of an individual*

The appearance of an animal is described as its phenotype. The dominant characteristic simply refers to one of a pair of alleles that is actually expressed. The gene that is not expressed is described as recessive. The word homozygous also refers to a pair of alleles, but in this case the alleles are identical to each other.

9 Exotic pets and wildlife

1. A *The animal that has a gestation period of over 60 days and
young that are born with fur and eyes open is the guinea pig*
The rat has a gestation period of about 20–22 days. The
gestation period for the Syrian hamster is 15–18 days, and
slightly longer for the Russian or Chinese hamsters. The
gerbil has a gestation period of between 24 and 26 days.

2. D *Rabbits do not have pads on their feet*
Rabbits have thick fur on the soles of the feet and between
the toes. The other species have pads on their feet.

3. D *Ferrets reach sexual maturity at 6–9 months*
This varies a little, as they are seasonal breeders. The main
breeding season is between February/March and September, so
a young ferret born in April/May may not start being sexually
active until almost a year old.

4. D *The gestation period of the chinchilla is 111 days*

5. C *The ferret is an induced ovulator*
The queen and the rabbit are also induced ovulators.

6. B *Budgerigars can be sexed by the colour of the cere*
In the cock birds the cere is blue, in the hen it is brown.
    Most birds are not sexually dimorphic (that is, there are no
distinct physical characteristics that distinguish males from
females), and a blood test or laparoscopy has to be performed
for sexing.

7. A *The normal temperature for a rabbit is 38.0–40°C
(100.4–104°F)*

8. D *The canary belongs to the passeriformes*
The passeriformes are perching birds, and the order also
includes finches and thrushes.
    The galliformes include chickens, pheasants and quail.
Parrots and budgerigars are psittaciformes, and the strigiformes
are owls.

9. C *Guinea pigs should be housed at temperatures between 12 and
20°C*

10. D *A tropical fish tank is usually kept between 21 and 29°C*
The exact temperature depends on the particular species of fish
being kept.
Coldwater tanks should be kept at temperatures up to 21°C.

11. A *The tortoise is ectothermic*
Ectothermic means cold blooded. Another term occasionally
used for ectothermic animals is poikilothermic.
Warm-blooded animals are endothermic.

12. C *Dwarf hamsters can be kept as pairs*
Dwarf hamsters can be kept in pairs if they are introduced
when young.
Golden or Syrian hamsters (these are the same breed) are
solitary animals, and will fight except when breeding.

13. D *A mouse can be picked up by the tail*
This should never be done to gerbils, as the skin sloughs quite
easily. Gerbils should be picked up by the base of the tail
providing they are supported under the body or, if tame, picked
up with cupped hands.
Rats are too heavy to be picked up by the tail. They should
be picked up around the thorax, with a thumb under the jaw to
prevent biting if needed.
Hamsters should be picked up by grasping the loose skin
around the neck and back and lifting. It is important to get
a good hold, as they can often swivel round and bite.
Alternatively, a small cloth can be used to hold the animal.

14. B *The best technique for the restraint of a guinea pig is to grasp
around the shoulders with a thumb under the jaw, and support
the hindlegs*
The thumb placed under the jaw prevents the animal from
being able to bite.

15. C *Rabbits can be calmed by covering the eyes*
When handling rabbits they can be scruffed, but the ears should
never be included.
Turning rabbits onto their backs often makes them panic
even more, so this is not to be recommended.

16. D *Mediterranean tortoises are mainly herbivorous*
The different species of chelonia have very different nutritional requirements. The box tortoises are more omnivorous than the Mediterranean species, and as youngsters need a mainly carnivorous diet. Turtles and terrapins are also carnivores.

17. B *The term dysecdysis is used to refer to difficulty sloughing the skin*
Dyschezia means difficulty passing faeces. Stomatitis is an inflammatory condition of the mouth, in reptiles sometimes referred to as 'mouth rot'. White spot is a parasitic condition fairly commonly seen in fish.

18. A *Of the species listed, the ferret may require vaccination*
Ferrets can be vaccinated if necessary against distemper. The other pet that should be vaccinated is the rabbit, which can be protected against myxomatosis and viral haemorrhagic disease.

19. D *A female guinea pig is called a sow*
A jill is a female ferret, a doe is a female rabbit, and a pen is a female swan.

20. B *Hamsters are nocturnal animals*
Gerbils are diurnal, whereas rats and mice can be active at any time.

10 Anatomy and physiology

Cells, tissues and cell chemistry

1. B *In intracellular fluid, sodium and chloride concentrations are low, potassium is high*
In the cell membrane of most cells there is a protein that acts as a sodium–potassium pump. This pushes sodium out of cells against its concentration gradient, and exchanges the ions for potassium ions. This is an active process, and requires energy.

The difference in composition between intracellular and extracellular fluid is essential for the body to operate normally. It is particularly important for the normal functioning of the nerve and muscle cells.

2. A *Salt is an example of an electrolyte*
An electrolyte is any substance which when placed in solution will separate into an anion and a cation. In solution salt dissociates into sodium and chloride ions:

$$NaCl \rightleftharpoons Na^+ + Cl^-$$

Glucose will dissolve in water, but remains as an entire molecule. Starch and fat do not dissolve.

3. C *Ribosomes are the organelles responsible for protein synthesis*
Mitochondria contain enzymes and produce energy for the cell.

The Golgi apparatus is involved with secretion, and lysosomes are vacuoles within the cytoplasm that contain digestive enzymes.

4. B *If a cell is placed in a hypertonic solution of sodium chloride, water will move out of the cell by osmosis*
Cell membranes are semipermeable membranes that allow water to pass through them but prevent other substances from doing so. If a solution of higher concentration is placed outside a cell, water will move by osmosis from the area of lower osmotic pressure to the area of higher osmotic pressure – that is, from inside the cell to outside. This will continue until the osmotic pressures are equalized.

5. C *The sex cells divide by meiosis to produce the sperm and ova*
Meiotic division results in the formation of four daughter cells. They are not identical to each other, or to the parent cell, and only contain half the genetic information of the parent cell.

Most cells in the body divide by mitosis. Nerve cells are the exception, since once formed they do not divide. Mitosis results in the development of two daughter cells that are identical to each other and to the parent cell.

6. A *Iron is needed within the body for haemoglobin, the pigment in red blood cells*
Haemoglobin is the part of the red blood cells that is necessary for the cells to be able to carry oxygen and carbon dioxide.
The mineral needed for bones and teeth, normal nerve and muscle function and blood clotting is calcium.

7. C *The average quantity of fluid lost per day by a healthy animal is 40–60 ml/kg*
Losses arise through respiration and sweat, urine and faeces. Sweat and respiratory losses account for 20 ml/kg, urinary losses are usually about 20 ml/kg and faecal losses vary from 0–20 ml/kg.

8. A *The bladder contains transitional epithelium*
This type of stratified epithelium can be stretched, which gives the bladder its ability to increase or decrease in size depending on the quantity of urine it contains.

9. D *The mediastinum contains the heart, aorta, vena cava, azygos vein and oesophagus*
The mediastinum contains all the organs that lie in the centre of the thoracic cavity.

10. D *An anabolic reaction occurs when simple substances combine together to form more complex molecules and this process uses up energy*
The opposite to this type of 'building up' reaction is catabolism, in which larger molecules are broken down into smaller ones with the release of energy.

11. B *Areolar tissue is another name sometimes used for loose connective tissue*
Loose connective tissue is usually present in the body as a 'packing material' between different tissues. Dense connective tissue is found where there is a greater need for strength, such as the sclera of the eye, or tendons and ligaments. Fluid connective tissues include blood and lymph, and the solid connective tissues are bone and cartilage.

12. C *Hyaline cartilage is found on the articular surfaces of bones*
The pinna of the ear and the epiglottis both contain elastic
cartilage, and the intervertebral discs are made of
fibrocartilage. The different types of cartilage reflect the
prevalence of different fibres within their structure, and the
different arrangement of the fibres.

The skeletal system

1. C *The patella is a sesamoid bone*
Sesamoid means seed, and sesamoid bones are small seed-like
bones that form in the tendons of muscles. The patella is the
largest sesamoid bone in the body, but there are many others,
such as the two fabellae in the tendons of origin of the
gastrocnemius muscle.
  The carpal bone, vertebra and phalanx are all examples of
bones that form by endochondral ossification. A cartilage
precursor is formed first, and is then gradually replaced
by bone.

2. A *New bone is synthesized by osteoblasts*
Osteocytes are resting or old osteoblasts found within tiny holes
in bone. Chondrocytes produce cartilage, and osteoclasts are
cells that break down bone to release calcium and
phosphate ions.

3. B *The epiphysis of a bone is the end of the bone*
The midshaft of a bone is the diaphysis, and the growth plate is
called the physis.

4. A *The carpal bone forms by endochondral ossification*
The parietal bone, like the other flat bones of the skull, forms
by intramembranous ossification. The patella is an example of
a sesamoid bone, which forms in the tendon of a muscle at a
point of wear. The os penis is part of the splanchnic skeleton,
which consists of bones that develop in tissues and are
unconnected to the rest of the skeleton.

5. B *The carnassial teeth of the dog are the fourth upper premolars
and the first lower molars*

6. A *The unpaired bone in the skull that surrounds the foramen
magnum is the occipital bone*
The foramen magnum is the hole through which the spinal cord
passes to reach the brain. The tympanic and zygomatic bones
are both paired, and form the zygomatic arches on each side of
the skull.
  The vomer is unpaired but lies in the midline, forming part of
the floor of the nasal cavity.

7. C *There is a meniscus in the temporo-mandibular joint*
Menisci are fibrocartilaginous pads that sit between the bones of a joint. As well as one in the temporo-mandibular joint, there are two menisci in each stifle joint. These act as shock absorbers and improve the congruity between the femur and the tibia.

8. C *The lumbar vertebrae have short spinous processes and long transverse processes that are directed ventrally and cranially*
The cervical vertebrae are small box-like vertebrae with short spinous processes and short transverse processes. Their shape allows flexibility of the neck.
    Thoracic vertebrae have very long spinous processes and relatively short transverse processes. The sacral vertebrae are fused in the dog and cat, and articulate with the ilium of the pelvis on each side.

9. C *Foetal bones start to ossify about 6–7 weeks through gestation*

10. D *There are 13 thoracic vertebrae in the dog*

11. A *The glenoid cavity is found within the shoulder joint*
The glenoid cavity is the space formed by the concavity of the articular surface of the scapula.

12. B *The cranial cruciate ligament is an important structure within the stifle*
This ligament is often damaged if the stifle is twisted forcefully. This results in a laxity in the stifle joint such that the tibia is able to move cranially relative to the femur. Injury to the cranial cruciate ligament is painful, and if ruptured usually requires surgery to replace the ligament and restore joint stability.

13. B *The sacrum is not part of the appendicular skeleton*
The skeleton can be divided into two parts: the appendicular skeleton, which includes all the bones of the limbs, and the axial skeleton, which comprises the skull, vertebrae, ribs and sternum.

14. D *The inervertebral disc is an example of an amphiarthrosis*
Amphiarthroses are cartilage joints where there is a little movement. Joints that have a wider range of movement, such as the stifle, are synovial joints. The articulations between the ribs and the vertebrae are also synovial joints. The skull sutures are immovable fibrous joints.

15. C *The holes formed by adjacent vertebrae through which the spinal nerves emerge are called the intervertebral foramina*
The foramen magnum is the large hole in the occipital bone of the skull through which the spinal cord passes. The nutrient foramen is the name given to the hole found in many bones that allows blood vessels to reach the bone marrow.

The vertebral canal is the hole in the centre of the vertebrae through which the spinal cord runs.

16. A *The bone that forms the point of the hock is the os calcis*
This bone has several names; it is also called the tuber calcis, the calcaneus or the fibular tarsal bone.

The anconeal process is found on the ulna at the proximal end of the notch, where it articulates with the humerus.

The tibial tuberosity is found at the proximal end of the tibial crest, and is where the tendon of quadriceps femoris has its insertion. The patella is the sesamoid bone found within the tendon of quadriceps.

17. B *The dental formula of an adult cat is I 3/3, C 1/1, PM 3/2, M 1/1*
I 3/3, C 1/1, PM 4/4, M 2/3 is the dental formula of an adult dog.
I 3/3, C 1/1, PM 3/3 is the dental formula of a puppy.
I 3/3, C 1/1, PM 3/2 is the dental formula of a kitten.

The muscular system

1. C *Epaxial muscles are found above the transverse processes of the vertebrae*
The muscles below the transverse processes are the hypaxial muscles.

2. B *Contraction of the gastrocnemius muscle causes flexion of the stifle and extension of the hock*
The gastrocnemius crosses the caudal aspect of both the stifle joint and the hock joint, and therefore will affect both joints when it contracts. The line of pull across the stifle is not good, and so it is only a weak stifle flexor, but it is a strong hock extensor.

3. D *The palpebral muscles are striated muscles*
'Striated' is another name given to skeletal or voluntary muscle owing to the appearance of these cells under the microscope.
   The muscles of the small intestine and the arrector pili muscles are smooth or involuntary muscles controlled by the autonomic nervous system.
   Cardiac muscle is only found in the heart, and is quite different from either smooth or skeletal muscle.

4. B *Cardiac muscle undergoes spontaneous contractions*
Cardiac muscle is unique in structure and function. All cardiac muscle cells can contract spontaneously without the need for nervous stimulation. The contractions are, however, modified by the autonomic nervous system. Heart muscle, unlike skeletal muscle, is not easily fatigued, but in common with all muscle cells it does require energy to contract.

5. C *The aponeurosis in the ventral abdominal midline where the abdominal muscles fuse is called the linea alba*
The linea alba is the tendon sheet between the four paired abdominal muscles – the rectus abdominis, internal and external abdominal oblique and transversus abdominis.
   The prepubic tendon is the point of insertion for the rectus abdominis muscle in front of the pubis.
   The inguinal ring is a natural opening through the layers of abdominal musculature that allows blood vessels and nerves to leave the abdominal cavity and supply the hindlimbs.

6. C *The prime protractor of the forelimb is brachiocephalicus*
Contraction of brachiocephalicus causes the forelimb to be swung forward. This occurs in the non-weight bearing phase of the forelimb stride.

Biceps brachii is the prime elbow flexor, with brachialis acting as a secondary or weaker flexor.

Trapezius links the scapula to the thoracic vertebrae. Contraction causes slight elevation and rotation of the scapula.

7. B *Biceps femoris, semimembranosus and semitendinosis form the hamstrings*
The hamstrings act together to extend the hip and drive the body forward during locomotion.

8. B *Anterior tibial does not form part of the Achilles tendon*
The Achilles tendon is made of tendons that either have their insertion on or pass over the os calcis in the hock. The four tendons that contribute to its structure are the tendons of insertion of gastrocnemius, semitendinosis, biceps femoris and superficial digital flexor.

The anterior tibial is a muscle that runs down the cranial aspect of the tibia and crosses the cranial surface of the hock joint. It causes hock flexion.

9. D *The patella is found in the tendon of insertion of quadriceps femoris*
The patella is a sesamoid bone, which develops in the tendon of quadriceps femoris at the point where the tendon passes through the trochlear groove of the femur. It protects the tendon from the wear and tear it would receive at this site.

10. A *The muscle that has its origin on the thoracic vertebrae is trapezius*
Supraspinatus and infraspinatus have their origins above and below the spine of the scapula respectively, and insert on the humerus.

Triceps brachii has its origin on the humerus, and inserts on the olecranon of the ulna.

11. A *Latissimus dorsi is not an intrinsic muscle of the forelimb*
An intrinsic muscle is one that has both its origin and insertion on the same region of the body, for example, within the forelimb or within the head.

Brachialis, supraspinatus and triceps brachii all have their origins and insertions on the bones of the thoracic limb. Latissimus dorsi has its origin on the thoracic vertebrae and ribs, and its insertion on the medial humerus.

12. A *The adductor of the hindlimb is pectineus*
An adductor is a muscle that draws the limb medially.

Quadriceps femoris is a stifle extensor. The semimembranosus causes hip extension, and contraction of gastrocnemius results in hock extension and stifle flexion.

The integument

1. B *Mammary glands are modified apocrine glands*
Apocrine glands are found all over the body of the animal, and are more commonly referred to as sweat glands. There are also more specialized sweat glands found only on the pads which are called merocrine glands. Sebaceous glands are associated with hairs and produce sebum, which lubricates the hairs and gives the coat its water repelling quality.

2. C *The skin is not involved with vitamin E metabolism*
The skin is needed to keep the animal 'waterproof', and for fat storage.
   Vitamin D requires activation by exposure to ultra-violet light before it can be used by the body. This takes place in the skin.

3. A *Sebaceous glands originate from the epidermis*
Sebaceous glands are formed by epidermal cells growing downwards into the dermis to form a channel. The glands retain their connection with the epidermis so their secretions are able to reach the surface. Sebaceous glands produce sebum, an oily secretion needed to keep the skin and coat supple and flexible. It also helps with waterproofing and insulation of the skin, and carries pheromones.

4. C *The cerumen glands of the ear are sebaceous glands*
The cerumen glands are modified sebaceous glands, and produce a thicker secretion than most sebaceous glands. This is usually known as earwax, and helps to protect the external ear canal from infection.

5. D *The epidermis is made of stratified squamous epithelium*
Columnar epithelium is a single layered epithelium, usually found where absorption or secretion takes place. Transitional epithelium is a multilayered epithelium, which has the property of being able to be stretched. This is found lining the bladder. Mesothelium is used to refer to some of the simple squamous epithelia in the body, for example those lining body cavities.

6. C *Hair is not needed for vitamin D activation*
The hair coat is not involved with vitamin D activation, which takes place in the skin in the presence of sunlight.
   Hair can be raised by the contraction of the arrector pili muscles. The hairs trap a thicker layer of air against the body, which acts as an insulator and prevents the animal from losing body heat.

The colour markings of animals are used both for defence and for recognition. This is not the only cue that animals use to recognize each other, but it does seem to be an important factor within social groups.

There are specialized hairs with increased numbers of nerve endings that are involved with tactile sensations. These include the vibrissae or whiskers, and the cilia or eyelashes.

7. B *The tissue that forms the 'quick' of the claw is the dermis*
There is no single digital vein running through the claw, but many capillaries run within the dermal tissue beneath the hard epidermis that forms the outer tissue of the claw.

The coronary band is the area from which the claw grows under the claw fold.

8. A *Epidermal cells divide in the agranular or basal cell layers of the epidermis*
The newly formed cells then move up through the granular or parietal cell layer as the cells beneath continue to divide. They become flatter and lose their nuclei as they are pushed upwards, and finally form the outermost cornified or keratinized layer. The cells are then worn away from the skin's surface through wear and tear.

It takes about 30 days for cells to move from the basal cell layer to the top of the keratinized layer.

The respiratory system

1. B *Inspiration of air into the lungs is produced by contraction of the diaphragm*
The diaphragm is the main muscle of inspiration, and when it contracts it flattens out and enlarges the thoracic cavity. There is a small amount of negative pressure within the pleural cavities, and this causes the lungs to expand and draw in air.
    The abdominal muscles are only involved in respiration if the animal is under severe stress or in breathing difficulty, when they assist with expiration. Vertebral muscles are not involved in respiration, and there are no sternal muscles as such.

2. D *'Dead space' refers to the part of the respiratory tract that is not available for gaseous exchange*
The areas within the respiratory tract not available for gaseous exchange include the nasal chambers, pharynx, larynx, trachea, bronchi and bronchioles.

3. B *The 'tidal volume' is the volume of air inspired and expired during normal respiration*
The maximum amount of air that can be inspired and expired is the 'vital capacity'.
    The volume left in the lungs after normal expiration is the 'functional residual capacity' and the volume of air left in the lungs after forced expiration is called the 'residual volume'.

4. D *The order in which inspired air passes through the structures of the airways is: trachea, bronchi, respiratory bronchioles, alveolar ducts and alveoli*

5. A *The right lung has four lobes, the left has three*
Both lungs have cranial or apical lobes, middle or cardiac lobes, and caudal or diaphragmatic lobes. The right lung has an extra lobe between the middle and caudal lobes called the accessory or intermediate lobe.

6. C *Inspired air contains 21% oxygen*
The composition of air is 79% nitrogen, 21% oxygen, 0.03% carbon dioxide and 1% water vapour.

7. D *The sinus connected to the nasal chambers and lined with mucous membrane is the frontal sinus*
This is the only true sinus in the dog. There is also a maxillary sinus, but this is just a hollow within the maxilla, is not lined with mucous membrane and does not connect with the respiratory tract.

8. A *The term used to describe a fast respiratory rate is tachypnoea*
Tachycardia is a fast heart rate. Dyspnoea means difficulty breathing, and orthopnoea means that the animal is having such severe breathing difficulties that it has to remain sitting up with its elbows abducted in order to take in sufficient oxygen.

9. B *Gaseous exchange across the alveolar walls takes place by diffusion*
The respiratory gases simply diffuse from areas of high gas concentration to areas of low gas concentration.
Osmosis is the movement of water across a semi-permeable membrane from an area of low osmotic pressure to an area of high osmotic pressure.
Active transport systems involve the movement of substances against their concentration gradient – that is, from an area of low concentration to an area of high concentration.
Filtration is the movement of a liquid under pressure through a membrane such that water and small molecules can pass through, but larger molecules are kept behind.

10. A *The respiratory centres that control respiration are found in the hindbrain*
These control the basic respiratory cycle, but breathing can be modified due to the influence of higher areas in the brain. This occurs in voluntary breath holding, or when respiratory patterns change due to pain or fear.

Blood and the circulatory system

1. D *The cellular component of blood produced from a megakaryocyte is the thrombocyte*

A megakaryocyte is a large multinucleate cell found within the bone marrow.

Thrombocytes (platelets) are produced as small pieces of cytoplasm, which bud off from the cell and enter the circulation.

Erythrocytes and neutrophils are also produced within the bone marrow from myeloid tissue.

Lymphocytes are produced within the germinal centres of lymphoid tissue.

2. A *The innermost epithelial layer of the heart is called the endocardium*

The myocardium is the term for the heart muscle, and the epicardium is the serous membrane closely adherent to the outside of the myocardium. The pericardium is strictly made up of two parts: the epicardium; and a second serous membrane attached to a fibrous tissue layer, which envelops the heart. There is a tiny amount of pericardial fluid in the space between the two serous membranes, which is referred to as the pericardial cavity.

3. D *The branch of the aorta that supplies arterial blood to the head and neck is the common carotid artery*

The coeliac artery supplies the stomach, liver and spleen. The cranial mesenteric artery supplies the small intestine, and the subclavian artery on each side of the animal takes blood into the forelimb.

4. C *There is no lymphoid tissue within the bone marrow*

In the young animal the tissue in the marrow cavity is myeloid tissue, which produces all the cellular components of blood except the lymphocytes. As the animal gets older the myeloid tissue is largely replaced by fat, except within the heads of the long bones.

The spleen, lymph nodes and the thymus are all part of the lymphatic system, and all contain lymphoid tissue.

5. A *The monocyte is an agranulocyte*

This simply means that it does not contain granules within its cytoplasm.

Neutrophils, eosinophils and basophils all contain granules within their cytoplasm, which have different staining characteristics.

6. C *Deoxygenated blood is carried by systemic veins and pulmonary arteries*

The systemic veins return blood containing carbon dioxide and other waste products from the body to the heart. The pulmonary arteries take this blood from the heart to the lungs, where gaseous exchange takes place.

Oxygenated blood is therefore found in the systemic arteries and pulmonary veins.

7. C *Contractions are initiated in the sino-atrial node*

The sino-atrial node is a region within the right atrium of the heart. All cardiac muscle cells can undergo spontaneous contractions, but the cells in the sino-atrial node contract at a faster rate than anywhere else in the heart. Because of the electrical connections between adjacent cardiac muscle cells, the electrical activity triggered in this area is able to spread through the rest of the heart muscle.

From the sino-atrial node, the electrical activity is transferred through the atrio-ventricular node (which provides the electrical connection between atrial and ventricular tissue), down fibres called the Bundles of His (which lie in the septum between right and left ventricles), and finally to the Purkinje fibres within the walls of the ventricles.

8. C *The azygos vein is an unpaired vein*

The azygos vein collects venous drainage from the right side of the thorax, and empties either into the anterior vena cava or directly into the right atrium.

The external jugular veins run either side of the neck. There is a saphenous vein in each hindlimb, and the cephalic veins are found in the forelimbs. These veins all lie superficially and can be used for venepuncture in the dog and cat.

9. D *The name given to the caudal end of the thoracic duct, which receives lymph from the hindlimbs, lumbar region and abdominal organs, is the cisterna chyli*
The thymus is a lymphoid organ found in the mediastinum that is responsible for the development of one particular type of lymphocyte, called a T-cell.
 The right lymphatic duct collects lymph from the right forelimb and the right side of the head and neck. The tracheal ducts carry lymph from the head.

10. D *The hepatic portal vein links the intestinal capillary bed with the capillaries within the liver*
The hepatic portal vein is unusual in that it transfers blood from one capillary network to another. Most veins carry blood from capillaries to larger veins, eventually taking the blood to the vena cava.
 The caudal vena cava (or posterior vena cava) collects all the venous drainage from the abdomen and caudal parts of the body. The hepatic vein collects venous blood from the liver, and this then drains into the caudal vena cava. The cranial mesenteric artery supplies arterial blood to the small intestine.

11. D *Phagocytosis of bacteria is carried out by neutrophils*
Eosinophils are found in increased numbers in allergic responses and in severe parasitism. Basophils contain histamine and heparin, but are usually only present in the circulation in very low numbers. Lymphocytes are essential for the production of antibodies and for cell mediated immunity.

12. B *Eosinophils show characteristic red granules throughout the cytoplasm after staining*
Neutrophils do have granules in their cytoplasm, but these do not take up the stains well. Basophils have dark blue staining granules, and monocytes do not have any granules because they are agranulocytes.

13. B *The valve that separates the left atrium and left ventricle in the heart is the mitral valve*
The tricuspid valve is found between the right atrium and right ventricle. The pulmonic valve lies at the junction between the right ventricle and the pulmonary artery, and the aortic valve separates the left ventricle and the aorta.

14. A *The popliteal lymph node can be palpated caudal to the stifle joint*
The accessory axillary lymph node is located on the side of
the thorax close to the axilla, but is not always present. The
superficial inguinal lymph node is found in the groin on each
side, and the parotid lymph node is palpable just caudal to the
temporo-mandibular joint by the base of the ear.

15. C *Antibodies are produced by B-lymphocytes*
T-cells are also a type of lymphocyte, but these do not produce
antibodies. They are involved with cell-mediated immunity.
    Neutrophils and monocytes are phagocytes, and help to
remove bacteria and cellular debris.

The digestive system

1. A *Bile does not contain enzymes to help fat digestion*
However, bile is necessary for normal fat digestion. It contains
bile salts, which emulsify the fats or break them up into small
droplets so that the lipases found in the pancreatic and
intestinal juices can work on the fat molecules.

As well as bile salts, bile contains bile pigments such as
bilirubin, produced from the breakdown of haemoglobin, and
electrolytes. Bile is produced by the liver and stored in the
gall bladder until needed.

2. B *Fatty acids can be absorbed into the lacteals and enter the
blood stream via the lymphatics*
Fatty acids can also be absorbed directly into the blood stream,
although the majority enter the lacteals.

Glucose and amino acids are absorbed into the blood
capillaries, and are then carried via the hepatic portal vein to the
liver.

Fibre is neither digested nor absorbed, but passes through the
intestines unchanged.

3. A *Chyme is the mix of food, mucus and enzymes produced in the
stomach*
The milky fluid within the thoracic duct is called chyle. The
enzyme used to break down fats is lipase, and the exocrine
secretion produced by the pancreas is called pancreatic juice.

4. D *The order in which food passes through the sections of the
small intestine is: duodenum, jejunum and ileum*

5. B *Villi are found within the small intestine*
The villi are finger-like projections of the mucosa, which
increase the surface area over which nutrients can be absorbed
into the blood stream and lacteals.

The stomach mucosa is thrown into folds called rugae.

The rectum and colon have a larger diameter than the small
intestine, but do not have villi.

6. C *The liver does not store fat*
The liver is an extremely important organ, with many
functions. These include deamination of protein metabolites,
storage of minerals such as iron and copper, manufacture of
plasma proteins, generation of heat, elimination of sex
hormones, fat metabolism, formation of bile, carbohydrate
metabolism and storage of some vitamins.

7. B *The tongue is not made of smooth muscle*
The tongue consists of striated or skeletal muscle, which allows
the animal to move food around the mouth to assist with
chewing and swallowing. It is also helpful for lapping and
grooming. In addition, the tongue carries many sensory
receptors. It is very important as an area for water evaporation
and heat loss through panting, particularly for dogs.

8. B *The enzyme amylase is needed to digest carbohydrates*
Fats are broken down by lipases, and proteins by proteases.
Vitamins are not digested, but absorbed intact.

9. B *Bile is released from the gall bladder under the action of the*
hormone secretin
Secretin is produced by cells in the small intestine whenever
food enters the duodenum. It causes both bile and pancreatic
juice to be released so that the food can be digested.
  Gastrin is produced by the stomach. This stimulates the
goblet cells in the stomach wall to secrete hydrochloric acid.
  Pepsin is an enzyme secreted by the stomach and digests
proteins.
  Renin is a hormone released by the kidney when blood
pressure falls, and is involved in the restoration of normal
blood pressure.

10. A *The region that is common to both the digestive tract and the*
respiratory tract is the pharynx
The pharynx is divided into two parts by the soft palate: the
naso-pharynx and the oro-pharynx.
  The larynx is part of the respiratory system, and controls
airflow into the trachea.
  The Eustachian tube connects the middle ear to the
nasopharynx. It is opened during swallowing, which allows
pressure within the middle ear to equilibrate with environmental
pressure.
  The oesophagus links the pharynx with the stomach.

11. D *The fold of connecting peritoneum that links the stomach to the*
body wall is called the omentum
The mesentery links the small intestine to the body wall.
Ligaments are smaller cords of peritoneum that link organs.
  For example, the ovarian ligament lies between the ovary and
kidney. The parietal peritoneum is the peritoneum lining the
inside of the abdominal and pelvic cavities.

The urinary system

1. A *The area of the bladder where the ureters enter is called the trigone*
The trigone is a small triangular area cranial to the neck of the bladder on the dorsal surface.

The apex or vertex of the bladder is the most cranial part of the bladder. The body forms the majority of the bladder between the apex and the neck.

2. B *Some drugs are actively secreted into the proximal convoluted tubule*
Penicillins are one class of drug where this occurs, which means that they are useful antibiotics for renal and urinary tract infections.

Glucose is reabsorbed by the kidney tubule, but this takes place in the proximal convoluted tubule and not in the distal convoluted tubule.

Amino acids (like glucose) are useful substances for the body to conserve, and so are reabsorbed in the proximal convoluted tubule.

The kidney is very important in the regulation of pH within the body. As subtle changes in pH occur, bicarbonate and hydrogen ions are excreted or reabsorbed.

3. D *The function of the loop of Henle in the renal tubule is to excrete sodium and chloride ions to set up the concentration gradient between the cortex and the medulla of the kidney*
The loop of Henle is essential for setting up the concentration gradient within the kidney tissues. This is needed so that water will be drawn out of the collecting duct and the urine will be concentrated.

There is no net concentration of the urine within the loop of Henle. Although water is excreted in the descending limb, sodium and chloride are excreted in the ascending limb, which means that the fluid reaching the end of the loop of Henle is no more concentrated than that at the start of the loop.

Electrolyte balance takes place in the distal convoluted tubule.

4. A *Filtration of blood by the kidney takes place in the glomerulus*
Blood is filtered by passing it through a fine meshwork of capillaries so that water and small molecules and ions are squeezed through the basement membrane into Bowman's capsule. The fluid then passes into the proximal convoluted tubule.

5. A *The main function of the proximal convoluted tubule is reabsorption*
The proximal convoluted tubule reabsorbs substances useful to the body, such as amino acids, glucose and water.
   Potassium and sodium balance takes place in the distal convoluted tubule. Concentration of the urine occurs in the distal convoluted tubule and collecting duct, and the concentration gradient is set up by the loop of Henle.

6. D *Protein is not normally found in urine*
Water, electrolytes and urea are always found in urine.

7. C *Aldosterone controls sodium reabsorption in the distal convoluted tubule*
Aldosterone is a mineralocorticoid produced by the adrenal cortex. It acts on the kidney to increase sodium reabsorption. The sodium ions are exchanged for potassium ions in the distal convoluted tubule.

8. D *The normal pH for canine urine is 6.5*
The pH for carnivore urine is usually acidic. Feline urine is usually slightly more acidic than canine urine, with a pH of about 6. High pH levels can indicate the presence of bacteria.

9. B *The indentation in the side of the kidney where the renal artery and vein enter is called the hilus*
The cortex is the outer layer of the kidney where the glomeruli are found, and the medulla is the more central area where the sodium and chloride concentrations are high. The loops of Henle and collecting ducts extend into the medulla. The area where urine collects before being carried to the bladder via the ureter is the renal pelvis.

10. C *Anti-diuretic hormone acts on the collecting duct*
Anti-diuretic hormone (ADH) from the posterior pituitary acts on the collecting duct and distal convoluted tubule to make these parts of the tubule permeable to water. The concentration gradient through the renal tissues draws water out, and so results in the urine remaining within the collecting duct becoming concentrated.

The reproductive system

1. **A** *Testosterone is produced by the interstitial cells (Cells of Leydig) in the male*
The Sertoli cells synthesize oestrogen and nutrients for the sperm. Spermatogenic cells produce the sperm, and the anterior pituitary releases interstitial cell stimulating hormone, which is needed for the production of testosterone.

2. **B** *The order in which the sperm pass through the male genital tract is: seminiferous tubules, epididymis, deferent duct and urethra*

3. **C** *The mesometrium is associated with the uterus*
The broad ligament is a double fold of peritoneum that links the epithelium covering the reproductive tract with the parietal peritoneum. The part of the broad ligament associated with the ovary is the mesovarium, and the section associated with the uterine tube is called the mesosalpinx.

4. **C** *The accessory glands in the tom cat are the prostate and the bulbo-urethral glands*
The accessory glands add secretions to the sperm to produce semen. The fluids contain nutrients for the sperm, and increase the volume of the ejaculate. The dog only has one accessory gland, the prostate gland.

5. **D** *The order in which the ovum passes through the female reproductive tract is: infundibulum, uterine tube, uterine horn and uterine body*

6. **B** *The epididymis is where the sperm are stored*
During their time in the epididymis, the sperm undergo maturation. If they have not had time to mature, they are less able to fertilize an ovum.
   The sperm are produced in the seminiferous tubules by spermatogenic cells. Nutrients for the sperm are also produced in the tubules by Sertoli cells. Testosterone is produced by interstitial cells, or cells of Leydig, which lie between the seminiferous tubules.

7. **C** *An animal in which only one testis descends is described as cryptorchid*
The term cryptorchid is used to describe animals in which one or both testes are retained. These animals are not sterile, but a

retained testis will produce fewer sperm than normal since it is at a higher temperature than it would be in the scrotal sac. This can result in the development of tumours. Retained testes should therefore be removed before tumours develop.

Monorchidism is quite rare, and means that the animal only develops one testis. It is not advisable to breed from either monorchid or cryptorchid animals, as there is thought to be an inherited component to these conditions.

Orchitis means inflammation of the testis.

8. C *An animal that usually produces a litter of several young is described as being multiparous*
Polyoestrous animals are those that have several oestrous cycles within one breeding season. Multigravid animals are those than have been pregnant before, whereas a primigravid animal is pregnant for the first time.

9. D *The spermatic cord consists of the deferent duct, blood vessels, nerves, cremaster muscle and vaginal tunic*

10. D *A bitch will not allow herself to be mounted during proestrus*
During proestrus a bitch will show vulval swelling and a bloody discharge and will engage in courtship play, but she is not ready to allow mating until oestrus itself.

11. B *The hormone responsible for the signs and the behaviour changes seen in oestrus is oestrogen*
Oestrogen is produced by the developing follicles, and blood levels reach a maximum immediately prior to ovulation. It causes changes in the uterus that result in the bloody discharge and the flirting and mating behaviours seen in proestrus and oestrus.

Progesterone is only released once ovulation has taken place, as it is produced by the corpus luteum. This stops the mating behaviour, and results in the preparation of the uterus for implantation by the fertilized ovum. It is needed during pregnancy to maintain the correct environment for the developing embryo, and to prevent the animal ovulating while pregnant.

Follicle stimulating hormone is produced by the anterior pituitary, and this stimulates resting follicles to start the maturation process. Luteinizing hormone (LH) is the trigger for ovulation and the development of the corpus luteum. LH release is stimulated by the high oestrogen levels present just before ovulation occurs.

12. B *Colostrum does not contain more lactose than milk*
Colostrum is the first milk produced, and contains more protein than milk because it is rich in the immunoglobulins or antibodies needed by the young for protection until their own immune system is developed fully.

13. B *Oestrus in the bitch lasts between 7 and 10 days*

14. C *The bitch is a spontaneous ovulator and is monoestrous*
The bitch does not require mating in order to ovulate, and only shows one oestrus per breeding season. The queen on the other hand is an induced ovulator, and the stimulus of mating is needed to trigger the release of luteinizing hormone and ovulation. The queen is also seasonally polyoestrous. There are only certain times of the year in which she will breed, but during each breeding season she will come into oestrus several times.

15. A *The developing Graafian follicles within the ovary produce oestrogen*
Progesterone is produced only after ovulation has taken place, and is formed by the corpora lutea. Luteinizing hormone and follicle stimulating hormone are both produced by the anterior pituitary.

16. B *The placenta is formed from the allantois and the chorion*
The allantois, chorion and amnion are membranes that surround the embryo during its development.
   The amnion is a fluid-filled sac that cushions the embryo during pregnancy and birth. Often this does not rupture until after birth.
   The allantois is a second sac, which lies outside the amnion and is continuous with the gut of the foetus. Initially it only contains waste products from the foetus, but once the placenta is formed it is involved in the exchange of nutrients and waste products between the mother and the foetus.
   The chorion is the outermost tissue layer that surrounds the foetus, amnion and allantois, and this fuses with the outer layer of the allantois to form the allanto-chorion. It is this joint layer that forms the placenta.

17. A *Luteinizing hormone is produced by the anterior pituitary*

18. C *Pseudocyesis is another term for a false pregnancy*
Another name for a false pregnancy is phantom pregnancy.
    An animal that has sexual characteristics of both sexes is
called either an intersex or a hermaphrodite.
    Female animals do not stop their oestrous cycles as they get
older. There is no animal equivalent to the menopause in humans.

19. D *Oestrus in the bitch can be detected by using any of the
techniques*
The behaviour of the bitch changes once she comes into
oestrus, and at this time most bitches will allow the male to
mount. This is not always very reliable as a detection method,
since nervous bitches may not let a male mate them even when
they are in oestrus.
    Progesterone testing is used fairly frequently for oestrus
detection. Prior to ovulation progesterone levels are practically
zero, but once a corpus luteum is formed then progesterone is
released and blood concentrations increase. A bitch should
therefore be blood tested every 2 days in the week prior to an
expected oestrus. Detection of progesterone is a definite sign that
the bitch has ovulated and should be mated as soon as possible.
    Vaginal smears are also used as a means for testing for
oestrus. In proestrus, smears taken from the vagina contain
many red blood cells and few other cells. Once a bitch enters
oestrus, the numbers of red blood cells decline, and many
cornified cells without nuclei are seen.

20. D *The acrosome in the head of each sperm contains enzymes to
allow penetration of the ovum*
The head of the sperm also contains the nucleus of the cell.
Many mitochondria are found in the midpiece of the sperm,
which produces the energy needed to drive the tail. Nutrients
for the sperm are obtained from Sertoli cell secretions and the
seminal fluid produced by the accessory glands.

The nervous system

1. C *Myelin is made of the cell membranes of Schwann cells, which wrap around the axons of most neurones*
The axons and Schwann cells are surrounded by a connective tissue sheath – the neurilemma.

   Nerves are made of bundles of neurones bounded by a connective tissue nerve sheath.

2. B *Sympathetic neurones are carried by thoracic and lumbar spinal nerves*
Autonomic neurones only leave the central nervous system with specific spinal and cranial nerves. Sympathetic neurones are carried by the thoracic and lumbar nerves, and parasympathetic neurones by the cranial and sacral nerves.

3. D *The vagus nerve (cranial nerve X) supplies the thorax and abdomen with parasympathetic neurones*
Parasympathetic neurones only leave the central nervous system with cranial and sacral nerves. In order for parasympathetic neurones to reach the thorax and cranial abdomen, the neurones are carried by the vagus nerve, which runs down from the head, through the neck and into the thorax and abdomen.

   The facial nerve (cranial nerve VII) and the glossopharyngeal nerve (cranial nerve IX) also carry parasympathetic neurones, but these have their effects within the head region and cause lacrimation and salivation.

4. B *The parasympathetic nervous system causes increased gut movement*
The parasympathetic nervous system is responsible for many of the 'emptying functions' of the body, including defecation, urination and gastro-intestinal tract movement.

   The sympathetic nervous system produces what is known as the 'flight or fight response' – the heart rate is increased, there is peripheral vasoconstriction as blood is redirected to essential tissues, the hair stands on end and the pupils dilate as the body is prepared for action.

5. C *The tissues that overlie the central nervous system are called the meninges*
There are three tissue layers that form the meninges: the dura mater, a tough fibrous outer layer; the arachnoid mater, a web-like layer with cerebrospinal fluid between the strands of tissue; and the pia mater, a fine vascular layer that is closely adherent to the central nervous tissue lying beneath.

6. A *The withdrawal reflex is a spinal reflex*
It is also an unconditional reflex, as it is repeatable in different individuals and even in different species. Conditional reflexes are reflexes that have to be learnt, since the stimulus and response are not directly related.

The withdrawal reflex is a simple reflex, using only a pathway to and from the spinal cord. Complex reflexes involve input from higher areas of the central nervous system.

7. C *The cauda equina refers to the spinal nerves that extend from the caudal end of the spinal cord and continue to run within the vertebral canal*
When it was first dissected out this part of the nervous system was thought to resemble a horse's tail, and so was given the Latin name cauda equina.

8. A *The third ventricle is found within the forebrain*
There are four ventricles within the brain. The two lateral and third ventricles lie within the forebrain, and the fourth ventricle is found in the hindbrain. There is no ventricle in the midbrain, just a small channel called the cerebral aqueduct.

9. B *The part of the brain responsible for balance and co-ordination is the cerebellum*
The cerebral hemispheres are where interpretation of the incoming information takes place, and where memory and learning occur.

The medulla oblongata is part of the hindbrain and is responsible for many reflex activities, including the control of the heart and respiration.

The midbrain controls other more complex reflexes, and is involved in passing impulses between the forebrain and the rest of the central nervous system.

10. A *Sympathetic neurones reach the head via the sympathetic chain*
Autonomic neurones only leave the central nervous system with certain nerves, and sympathetic neurones emerge with the thoracic and lumbar spinal nerves. Sympathetic neurones are needed within the head to produce several responses, including pupil dilation. Having left the thoracic and lumbar spinal nerves, these neurones link together to form the sympathetic chain, which lies parallel to the spinal cord but outside the vertebrae. It runs cranially from the thorax and abdomen to the neck and head.

11. B *A synapse is the junction between one neurone and another*
The nerve endings or endplates contain transmitter, which is released when an impulse reaches this part of the nerve cell. Dendrites are the cytoplasmic outgrowths that conduct impulses towards the cell body, and the axon is the process that carries impulses away.

12. A *The dorsal root of a spinal nerve consists of somatic sensory and autonomic sensory neurones*
Within the bony arch of the vertebrae, spinal nerves are divided into two parts: the dorsal root, which contains just sensory neurones; and the ventral root, which only contains motor neurones. The dorsal and ventral roots contain both somatic and autonomic neurones.

13. B *The cerebral hemispheres are responsible for special senses, memory and awareness, and the voluntary control of movement*
See answer to Question 9.

14. C *The dorsal root ganglion contains the cell bodies of sensory neurones*
The dorsal root of a spinal nerve contains only sensory neurones, and there is a region called the dorsal root ganglion where all the cell bodies are found. There is no ganglion in the ventral root, as the cell bodies of motor neurones are found within the grey matter of the central nervous system.

15. C *The trigeminal nerve is cranial nerve V*

The trigeminal nerve supplies the temporal and masseter muscles, and also carries sensory neurones.

Cranial nerve III is the oculomotor nerve, which controls most movements of the eye.

Cranial nerve IV is the trochlear nerve, which is also involved with eye movement.

Cranial nerve VII is the facial nerve, which supplies many of the muscles of facial expression, and carries parasympathetic neurones to the salivary and lacrimal glands. It also carries sensory neurones that convey the sense of taste.

The special senses

1. **B** *Cranial nerves VII and IX carry information about taste*
   These are the facial and glossopharyngeal nerves respectively.

2. **A** *Pupil constriction is called miosis, and is produced by parasympathetic stimulation causing contraction of circular smooth muscles*
   Pupil dilation is mydriasis, and is produced by sympathetic stimulation causing contraction of radial smooth muscles within the iris.

3. **B** *Changes in final head position are detected by the utricle and saccule*
   The utricle and saccule are the otolith organs, which detect head position relative to gravity. The semicircular canals are sensitive to head movement, and the cochlea responds to sound waves. The middle ear transfers sound waves from the outer ear to the cochlea.

4. **B** *The stapes bone leans against the oval window*
   The three small bones within the middle ear, the ossicles, transfer sound waves from the outer ear to the inner ear. The first bone, or malleus, leans against the inside of the tympanic membrane or ear drum. Sound waves cause vibrations in the membrane, and the malleus transfers these to the second bone, the incus, which in turn transmits the vibrations to the last bone, the stapes bone. Vibrations of the stapes bone cause the oval window to move, and the vibrations are passed into the perilymph on the other side of the membrane. The round window lies below the oval window, and also separates the middle and inner ear.

5. **D** *The uvea or uveal tract within the eye consists of the iris, ciliary body and choroid*
   These structures are continuous with each other, and are all highly vascular and pigmented.

6. **B** *Light is refracted at the interior and exterior surfaces of the cornea and at the anterior and posterior surfaces of the lens*
   Light is refracted or bent whenever it passes through a junction between transparent media of different densities. Therefore refraction occurs at the junctions between the air and the cornea, between the cornea and the aqueous humour, between the aqueous humour and the lens, and between the lens and the vitreous humour. The curvatures of the cornea and lens play a vital role in the production of a focused image on the retina.

7. D *The Organ of Corti detects different sounds*
This is the sensory region within the cochlea that enables an animal to hear and interpret different sounds.

8. A *Cranial nerve I carries the sense of smell*
Cranial nerve I, the olfactory nerve, is made of many individual neurones that pass directly through the mesethmoid bone (also called the ethmoid bone or cribriform plate) to the olfactory lobes of the brain.

Cranial nerve II is the optic nerve, which carries information about sight. Cranial nerve VIII is the vestibulo-cochlear nerve, which conveys information about hearing and balance. Cranial nerve X is the vagus, which has several functions, including the carriage of parasympathetic neurones to the thorax and abdomen.

9. A *The ciliary body contains smooth muscles that enable an animal to accommodate for close and distant objects*
The ciliary body is connected to the edges of the lens via the suspensory ligament or zonule. Relaxation of the muscles within the ciliary body causes the lens to be pulled flatter. This means that images of distant objects will be in focus. When the muscles contract, the tension in the suspensory ligament decreases, and the lens is allowed to bulge. This enables the animal to focus on close objects.

The conjunctiva is the mucous membrane that surrounds the globe. The iris lies in front of the lens, and contains smooth muscle that can dilate or constrict the pupil and thus control the amount of light entering the eye.

The retina contains the light-sensitive receptors, the rods and cones, which respond to the light that enters the eye.

10. D *The fluid found in the posterior compartment of the eye is vitreous humour*
Vitreous humour is a gel-like material found between the lens and the retina. It helps to maintain the shape of the globe, and allows light to reach the retina.

Lacrimal fluid is produced by the lacrimal gland, and washes over the surface of the cornea. Aqueous humour is found in the anterior compartment of the eye. The choroid is the vascular pigmented layer of tissue lining the inside of the globe.

The endocrine system

1. D *The hormone produced by the posterior pituitary is oxytocin*
Adrenocorticotrophic hormone (ACTH) and luteinizing
hormone are both produced by the anterior pituitary.
   Calcitonin, also sometimes called thyrocalcitonin, is
produced by the thyroid glands.

2. B *The kidney helps control water balance within the body under
the influence of anti-diuretic hormone*
Adrenocorticotrophic hormone stimulates the adrenal glands to
produce glucocorticoids and mineralocorticoids. Calcitonin and
parathyroid hormone (or parathormone) are involved in the
regulation of calcium balance within the body.

3. A *A hormone that does not affect the kidney is erythropoietin*
Erythropoietin is produced by the kidney, and acts on the bone
marrow to stimulate the maturation of red blood cells.
   Aldosterone causes the kidney to conserve sodium, and
antidiuretic hormone acts on the kidney to increase water
reabsorption.

4. B *Adrenaline causes peripheral vasoconstriction, tachycardia and
pupil dilation*
Adrenaline has actions very similar to the effects of the
sympathetic nervous system, producing the 'fight or flight'
response. It is released from the adrenal medulla in response to
stimulation by the sympathetic nervous system.
   The thyroid hormones are involved with metabolism, and in
excess do cause a tachycardia, but the other signs would not
occur.
   Cortisol is produced by the adrenal cortex in response to
stress. It acts to maintain blood glucose levels, and has an
anti-inflammatory effect.
   Insulin is released after eating, and it acts on most cells in the
body to enable them to take up glucose from the blood stream.

5. B *The endocrine gland found in the brain is the pituitary gland*
The pituitary gland is an extremely important endocrine gland
that produces many hormones. Some of these regulate the
production of other hormones within the body, while others
have direct actions on tissues.
   The hypothalamus does not produce hormones, but sends
nervous impulses to the pituitary gland, which cause specific

hormones to be released. The thalamus is an area of the brain that sends impulses from the cerebral hemispheres to the rest of the central nervous system. The thyroid glands are endocrine glands, but are not found in the brain. These lie in the neck either side of the midline in front of the trachea.

6. B *If calcium levels in the blood fall, parathyroid hormone is released*
Parathyroid hormone acts to raise blood calcium levels by stimulating calcium release from bone through increased osteoclast activity and also improving calcium uptake from the intestine.

Calcitonin is a hormone involved with calcium balance, but it has the opposite effect to parathyroid hormone. It stimulates bone production and encourages blood calcium levels to fall, and so is only released when blood calcium concentrations are high.

Vitamin D is not a hormone, and is provided in the diet. It is needed so that calcium in food can be absorbed by the intestine.

The thyroid hormones are not directly involved with calcium regulation.

7. C *The hormone that regulates sodium levels in the body is aldosterone*
When sodium ion concentrations fall, aldosterone is released from the adrenal cortex. It acts to increase sodium reabsorption in the body, particularly by the kidney.

Angiotensin causes vasoconstriction, which increases blood pressure and stimulates the release of aldosterone.

Cortisol is released in times of stress, increasing the availability of glucose for the brain by preventing other tissues from using it and stimulating gluconeogenesis by the liver.

8. A *Testosterone is formed by the interstitial cells in the testes*
Testosterone is needed for the normal development of sperm and for the development of the secondary sex characteristics in the male animal.

Oestrogen is produced by Sertoli cells within the testes, and interstitial cell stimulating hormone (ICSH) is produced by the anterior pituitary. ICSH enables the interstitial cells to produce testosterone.

9. B *Adrenocorticotrophic hormone is released from the anterior pituitary*
Adrenocorticotrophic hormone acts on the adrenal glands to stimulate production of the corticosteroids.

10. A *The adrenal medulla produces the hormone adrenaline*
Aldosterone and cortisol are produced by the adrenal cortex, and adrenocorticotrophic hormone is produced by the anterior pituitary.

11. C *The thyroid hormones T_3 and T_4 control metabolic rate*
Calcium balance is controlled by parathyroid hormone and calcitonin.
Sodium balance is regulated by aldosterone.
Stress reactions are mediated by the glucocorticoids.

12. C *Glucagon stimulates gluconeogenesis by the liver*
Glucagon is produced by alpha cells within the islets of Langerhans of the pancreas. It is released when blood glucose levels fall, and acts to increase glucose concentrations within the blood stream. Glucose is stored in the liver in the form of the polysaccharide glycogen. Glucagon stimulates the breakdown of glycogen to release glucose.
Insulin is produced by beta cells within the islets of Langerhans, and has the opposite effect. It acts to decrease blood glucose levels after eating by allowing glucose uptake into the cells of the body. It also stimulates the synthesis of glycogen.
The thyroid hormones increase metabolic rate, but do not directly affect glucose balance.

11 Medicines: pharmacology, therapeutics and dispensing

1. A *A product for external use should be dispensed in a coloured fluted bottle*
Plain bottles should be used for oral liquid medicines. Wide-mouth jars are suitable for dispensing creams, powders or granules.

Tablets and capsules are generally dispensed in pots with child-proof lids, although if the client has problems with this type of lid, screw tops can also be used. Envelopes or paper wallets should only be used for sachets, foil strips and blister packs.

2. A *Miotics such as pilocarpine cause pupil constriction*
Mydriatics cause pupil dilation. Local anaesthetics desensitize the surface of the eye to allow minor procedures to be carried out. Hypromellose drops are used to replace or add to natural lacrimal fluid production.

3. B *The dog would require three tablets*
First calculate the dose the dog would need:
$$\text{Dose} = \text{dose rate} \times \text{body weight}$$
$$= 0.5 \times 30 \text{ mg}$$
$$= 15 \text{ mg}$$
Then calculate the number of tablets needed:
$$\text{Number} = \text{dose/tablet strength}$$
$$= 15/5$$
$$= 3 \text{ tablets}$$

4. D *Antitoxin contains antibodies to a toxin*
Antitoxins and other types of antisera contain antibodies and, when given to an animal, provide instant protection against the toxin or disease. However, the antibodies do not last very long – a matter of a few weeks. Vaccines contain organisms that have been weakened so that they will stimulate an immune response but do not actually produce disease. Toxoids are very similar, except that they contain altered toxin. The immunity developed in this way is described as *active immunity*, and is much longer lasting. Boosters are simply repeat injections of a vaccine or toxoid needed to maintain the animal's level of immunity.

5. B *The only piece of information not legally required on the label is the name of the drug and dosage*
However, it is good dispensing practice to give this information on the label of all items dispensed by a veterinary surgery.

6. C *Buprenorphine (Vetergesic) is an analgesic*
An analgesic is a drug that provides pain relief. Buprenorphine is one of several opiate drugs that are derived from opium. Others include morphine and pethidine.
   Diazepam (Valium) is a tranquillizer.
   Doxapram (Dopram) is a respiratory stimulant that acts on the respiratory centre of the brain.
   Atropine sulphate is an anticholinergic and is often used as a premedicant drug. It counters parasympathetic effects such as salivation and intestinal movement during surgery.

7. D *Pentobarbitone is a Schedule 3 Controlled Drug*
The Controlled Drugs are all drugs that could be abused by people. There are five schedules of Controlled Drugs. Schedule 1 contains hallucinogens and drugs not used in the medical professions, such as cannabis. Schedule 2 contains most of the opiates, such as pethidine. Schedule 3 includes the barbiturates and buprenorphine. Schedule 4 covers diazepam, some other tranquillizers and some anabolic steroids. Schedule 5 includes medicines that only contain tiny quantities of the drugs included in Schedules 1 to 4, such as cough mixtures containing the opiate codeine.

8. B *P products may legally be supplied by pharmacists and veterinary surgeons*
Medicines are classified into four types by the Medicines Act 1968. GSL (General Sales List) products can be sold by anyone. P (Pharmacy) products can only by sold by pharmacists and veterinary surgeons. PML (Pharmacy and Merchant List) products can be sold by pharmacists, veterinary surgeons and certain saddlers and agricultural merchants. POM (Prescription Only Medicines) products may only be prescribed by a veterinary surgeon, doctor or dentist, and are supplied only through a veterinary surgery or pharmacy.

9. C *An antitussive will suppress coughing*
Anti-emetics prevent vomiting, anthelminthics are drugs that kill worms, and antibiotics have an antibacterial effect.

10. D *The abbreviation that means three times daily is tid*
bid means twice daily, po means per os (by mouth), pr means
per rectum (given rectally).

11. B *The volume of drug that should be drawn up is 0.5 ml*
First calculate the dose needed by the cat:
$$Dose = dose\ rate \times body\ weight$$
$$= 0.2 \times 5\ mg$$
$$= 1\ mg$$
Then calculate the volume needed:
$$Volume = dose/concentration$$
$$= 1/2\ ml$$
$$= 0.5\ ml$$

12. D *The supply, purchase and storage of Controlled Drugs is*
covered by The Misuse of Drugs Act 1971 (and Misuse of Drugs
Regulations 1985)
The Medicines Act 1968 provides legislation for the
classification, manufacture, importation and dispensing of all
medicinal products.

The COSHH Regulations are an addition to the Health and
Safety at Work Act 1974, and these cover the use and storage of
all chemicals within the workplace.

The Health and Safety at Work Act outlines the
responsibilities of employers and employees in the
maintenance of a safe workplace. It has to be reasonably safe,
both for those working there and for any other persons that may
enter the premises.

13. B *The dog will require 2 ml of the anaesthetic*
First calculate the dose needed by the dog:
$$Dose = dose\ rate \times body\ weight$$
$$= 10 \times 5\ mg$$
$$= 50\ mg$$
Then calculate the concentration of the drug.

Knowing that the definition of a % solution is that it
contains that number of grams of drug in 100 ml,
a 2.5% solution = 2.5 g in 100 ml.
Because 1 g = 1000 mg, this is the same as
$$2.5 \times 1000\ mg\ in\ 100\ ml$$
$$= 2500\ mg\ in\ 100\ ml$$
We need the answer in mg/ml, so divide by 100:
2500/100 = 25 mg in 1 ml, or 25 mg/ml

Finally, calculate the volume needed:
Volume = dose/concentration
= 50/25 ml
= 2 ml

14. B *POM and PML products should not be stored in the consulting room, because they should not be kept anywhere that members of the public have access to*

15. D *In a veterinary practice, P, POM and PML products should only be dispensed to animals under a veterinary surgeon's care*
These drugs should only be dispensed to clients for animals that have been seen within the last 6 months. They should not be given to clients for animals that have not been seen by the veterinary surgeon.

A pharmacist may sell P and PML products over the counter to anyone, but can only sell POM products upon receipt of a written prescription from a doctor, veterinary surgeon or dentist.

12 Laboratory diagnostic aids

1. A *A centrifuge would be needed in order to measure packed cell volume (PCV)*
The packed cell volume (PCV) is a measurement of the proportion of a blood sample that is made up of cells. This can only be measured by centrifuging the sample so that all the cells are packed closely together, with the plasma or serum lying on top.

Haemoglobin estimation either requires colour matching by eye, or the use of a colorimeter or biochemistry analyser. Red blood cell and platelet counts require the use of diluting fluids, a microscope and counting chamber – usually the Improved Neubauer Counting chamber. These counts can also be performed automatically.

2. D *Dehydration is characterized by increased PCV and increased plasma protein levels*
In dehydration there is a loss of the fluid fraction of blood, so all cells and biochemical parameters are increased. This is true providing there is no pathology other than fluid loss.

3. C *Variation in erythrocyte size on a blood smear is called anisocytosis*
Spherocytosis means that the cells are not biconcave, but more spherical in shape.

Poikilocytosis means that the cells vary from the normal circular shape.

Anisochromasia means that the cells are not uniformly pigmented, and that there is variation in their colour.

4. D *When present in urine, ascorbic acid can mask a positive glucose reaction on urine dipsticks*
Dogs are able to synthesize vitamin C (ascorbic acid) in the intestines. If too much is produced it is cleared from the body by the kidney, and so can appear in the urine of normal animals. It affects the tests for glucose measurements because it inhibits the enzymes on the stick tests and produces false negatives, and it increases values for glucose when Clinitest or Benedict's reagent are used, thus leading to false positives with these tests.

5. B *The specific gravity of urine from this dog is most likely to be between 1.006 and 1.025*
The history and blood results confirm that the dog is in chronic renal failure. This usually means that the animal is unable actively to concentrate or dilute its urine as the renal tubules are no longer functioning adequately. The concentration of the urine will therefore be the same as the concentration of a filtrate of plasma, usually between 1.010 and 1.012. This is referred to as the isosthenuric range.

6. D *The most likely haematological abnormality is a decreased platelet count*
An increase in platelet numbers or changes in the PCV would not affect an animal's clotting ability. However, lack of platelets would result in multiple small haemorrhages occurring as minor damage is done to small blood vessels. Normally a tear in a blood vessel wall causes the platelets to change structure slightly and become sticky, so that they clump together and plug the hole. The clotting cascade is then activated, and eventually fibrin is laid down to form a more permanent seal over the site. Without the clotting factors, the platelet plug only lasts for about 24 hours and then disintegrates.

7. A *Severe parasitism can result in an eosinophilia*
Parasitic infestations that have systemic effects on the body stimulate an increase in the numbers of circulating eosinophils. Eosinophilia is also seen in allergic responses, and as an idiopathic finding in some individual animals. There have also been suggestions that increased numbers of eosinophils are found in animals with rage syndrome.

8. C *The normal PCV for a cat is 24–45%*

9. A *A differential white blood cell count should be stained using Leishman's stain*
A differential white blood cell count requires the use of a stain that will allow the identification of all the white blood cells. In order to do this the dye must have two components; one dye to highlight alkaline areas, and a second to show the acidic areas. Romanowsky stains such as Leishman's stain contain methylene blue, which stains alkaline areas dark blue, and eosin, which stains acidic areas red. This enables the white blood cells to be distinguished and counted.

Gram's stain is used to distinguish between Gram-positive and Gram-negative bacteria.

Lugol's iodine can be used in Gram's stain, or on its own to locate undigested starch within faecal smears.

New methylene blue is used as a supra-vital stain to identify reticulocytes.

10. A *Urinary casts are produced within the kidney tubules*
These are made of protein that is deposited within the tubules. The tubules act as a mould, and the resulting solid cast contains whatever other substances were present in the tubule at the same time. This can include white blood cells, fats, or epithelial cells from the walls of the tubules. The different appearances of the casts can provide information about pathology within the kidney.

11. C *The normal red blood cell count for a dog is 5.5–8.5 $\times 10^{12}$/l*
The normal white blood cell count for a dog is
$6-18 \times 10^9$/l

12. D *The white blood cells that usually make up 5% of the differential count are monocytes*
Neutrophils account for between 60 and 70%, lymphocytes for between 15 and 20%, and basophils for less than 1% of the total white blood cell count.

13. A *White blood cell diluting fluid contains acetic acid to lyse the red blood cells*
Without the acid the whole field of view within the counting chamber would be packed with red blood cells, which would make the white blood cells hard to identify and count. The diluting fluid also often contains a dye, such as crystal violet or malachite green, to stain the white blood cells and make them easier to see.

14. B *In order to determine a differential white blood cell count, the minimum number of white blood cells that should be counted is 100*
However, it is more accurate if 200 cells can be counted.

15. A *The enzyme that provides most information about damage to liver cells is ALT*

ALT (alanine amino transferase) is an enzyme found within liver cells. In cats and dogs this is the only place it is found, so any increases in serum or plasma levels of this enzyme indicate that there is damage to the liver cells.

AST or aspartate amino transferase is another enzyme also found in liver cells. However it is not liver-specific and is also found in cardiac and skeletal muscle cells, so damage to any of these cells will result in an increase in blood levels.

Cholesterol is produced by the liver as a by-product of fatty acid metabolism. Levels can be elevated in liver disease but will also be raised in other conditions, such as hypothyroidism and diabetes mellitus, or if the animal has just eaten.

Bilirubin is a bile pigment, which is normally excreted via the gall bladder into the intestine and lost from the body in faeces. It is produced as a waste product from haemoglobin breakdown in the circulation, then processed by the liver and made into bile. High bilirubin levels in the blood stream can therefore arise in one of three ways – through increased red blood breakdown (haemolysis), liver disease, or failure of normal bile excretion into the intestine. An increase in blood levels therefore does not automatically indicate liver disease.

16. A *Alcoholic Sudan III is the stain used to detect undigested fats in faecal smears*

Lugol's iodine is used to detect undigested starch, and eosin shows up undigested muscle. Another dye used to detect muscle fibres is new methylene blue, which is also used to identify reticulocytes in blood smears.

17. D *Urine intended for bacterial studies should be preserved using boric acid*

Universal tubes containing boric acid are usually indicated by having a red cap.

Toluene is good for preserving urine for chemical examination. Formalin and thymol are good general-purpose preservatives, especially for examination of urinary sediments.

18. C *White cell casts in a urine sample collected via catheterization would indicate clinical disease*
White cell casts are only seen in disease conditions such as pyelonephritis or glomerulonephritis. Mucus and spermatozoa are common findings within the urinary tract, and transitional epithelial cells are often seen in urine samples from catheterized patients because the catheterization process displaces them from the walls of the urinary tract.

19. A *When using Leishman's stain, the undiluted stain should be left on the slide for 2 minutes*
It is then diluted using distilled water with pH 6.8, and left for over 10 minutes. The slide is then washed with distilled water and stood up to dry.

20. B *The total magnification of a microscope is calculated by multiplying the eyepiece magnification with the objective magnification*

21. C *A colorimeter measures the amount of light absorbed by a coloured solution*
Coloured solutions absorb a particular wavelength of light, and the amount of light that passes through the solution is compared with the light passing through a colourless solution so that the amount absorbed can be calculated.
    The intensity of the colour of the solution is related to the concentration of the solution. Therefore, if the absorption for a solution of unknown concentration is compared with the absorption of a solution of known concentration, the concentration of the unknown solution can be determined.

22. B *Before drawing off serum, blood should be allowed to clot for at least 30 minutes*
However, it should not be allowed to stand for longer than 2 hours before the serum is removed, as the clot starts to break down after this time.

23. D *The bacterium that needs to be stained using the Ziehl–Neelsen staining technique is Mycobacterium tuberculosis*
Mycobacterium tuberculosis is one of several bacteria that are described as being acid-fast. They are not stained easily using Gram's stain or methylene blue, but require this specialized staining technique to be viewed under the microscope.

24. D *A supra-vital staining technique has to be used to identify reticulocytes*
Supra-vital staining techniques involve culturing living cells with the stain, so that the dye is taken up into organelles. This technique is used for reticulocytes, immature red blood cells that still contain the remnants of organelles within their cytoplasm. The cells are cultured at 37°C with the dye for 30 minutes immediately after sampling, and a smear is then made in the same way as a blood smear is normally made.

The dyes that are used in this way are brilliant cresyl blue and new methylene blue, and both show the organelles as darker blue strands within the cytoplasm.

25. C *Bilirubin would be found in the urine of a dog suffering from obstructive jaundice*
In obstructive jaundice, there is obstruction to the normal outflow of bile from the gall bladder into the small intestine. Therefore, bile produced by the liver dams back into the circulation and blood bilirubin levels increase. This is seen clinically as jaundice. Eventually the bilirubin levels exceed the renal threshold, and bilirubin is found within the urine.

26. D *The bacteria that would appear as Gram-negative rods under the light microscope are Escherichia coli*
Streptococci and staphylococci are both Gram-positive cocci. The streptococci tend to form chains of organisms, and staphylococci are more likely to be found in clumps. Clostridia are also Gram-positive, but are short rods.

27. A *Struvite (ammonium triple phosphate) crystals usually appear like coffin lids*
Cystine crystals are usually hexagonal in appearance. Urates resemble thorn apples, and calcium oxalate crystals are octahedral and are often described as looking like envelopes when viewed through the microscope.

13 Elementary microbiology and immunology

1. C *The difference between Gram-negative and Gram-positive bacteria is that Gram-negative bacteria have an extra cell wall layer*
The extra layer possessed by Gram-negative bacteria is made of lipopolysaccharide (LPS), and is responsible for the different staining characteristics of Gram-negative bacteria compared with Gram-positive bacteria. It also confers some of the pathogenicity of Gram-negative bacteria.

Both Gram-negative and Gram-positive organisms can have flagella, though not all do, and there are pathogenic examples of both types of bacteria.

2. C *Bacteria reproduce by simple binary fission*
Bacteria divide by asexual division, in which the entire contents of a cell are duplicated and then divided equally into two cells. Mitosis is the equivalent type of cell division that takes place in the majority of animal cells.

Conjugation and spore formation are survival techniques used by some bacteria to overcome conditions that are not favourable to their survival. Conjugation occurs in some Gram-negative bacteria and involves the transfer of small pieces of genetic information from one cell to another. Spore formation is seen in some Gram-positive bacteria, and results in the development of a spore that is very resistant to disinfectants, heat and drying. Once conditions improve, the bacterium returns to its vegetative form and starts to reproduce normally again.

3. C *Structural components of all viruses include a protein capsid and nucleic acid*
Viruses are very simple organisms that only have to consist of a protein shell and their genetic information. The genetic code can be carried as either RNA or DNA. Some viruses are slightly more complex and in addition have other structures such as an envelope, but this is not seen in all types.

183

4. B *The bacterium that can form spores is Clostridium tetani*
Only certain Gram-positive bacteria can form spores, and these include the Clostridia and Bacillus species. The spores can remain dormant for long periods of time in the environment, until they encounter conditions that are favourable for growth again.

5. C *Exotoxins are produced by Gram-positive bacteria*
Exotoxins are substances produced and released by some Gram-positive bacteria. The toxins increase the organism's virulence or capability to produce disease, and they are quite easily destroyed by heat but can be very toxic. They are produced and released while the bacterium is still alive.
   Endotoxins are formed by Gram-negative bacteria. Endotoxin is the lipopolysaccharide layer of the cell wall, and so is only released once the bacterium dies. Endotoxins produce signs of shock when present in large quantities, but if only a small amount is present then the signs are of mild fever and malaise. They can withstand boiling, but are destroyed at temperatures over 120°C.

6. C *The term 'commensal' relates to bacteria that live in or on the host without causing harm*
Bacteria that are of benefit to the host are described as mutualistic.

7. D *The term used to describe curved bacteria is 'vibrios'*
Cocci are round bacteria, bacilli are rods and spirochaetes are spiral filaments

8. C *Deoxycholate citrate agar is a selective medium*
Deoxycholate citrate agar is used for the detection of Salmonella bacteria. Nutrient agar is a basic agar mix on which most bacteria will grow. Blood agar and chocolate agar contain the same basic nutrients as nutrient agar, but have had blood products added. They are sometimes called enriched media. These types of media are used for some fastidious bacteria that require additional nutrient factors.

9. D *Anaerobic conditions are required to grow Clostridia bacteria*

10. A *Viruses are measured in nanometres, nm (1×10^{-9} m)*
Bacteria are quite a bit larger, and are measured in micrometres, μm (1×10^{-6} m).

11. C *The term 'facultative anaerobe' is used to describe a bacterium that can grow in the absence of oxygen, but grows better when oxygen is available*
A bacterium with an absolute requirement for oxygen is an obligatory aerobe.
A bacterium that grows optimally without oxygen is an anaerobe.
A bacterium that grows best in minute quantities of oxygen is a microaerophile.

12. C *A toxoid contains antigen from a toxin*
A toxoid is something that mimics a toxin without causing the tissue damage a toxin would produce. It stimulates an immune response to the toxin and the development of antibodies. Antigen from a micro-organism is used within vaccines to stimulate an immune response to the organism.
Antitoxin contains antibodies to a particular toxin, and antiserum (sometimes called hyperimmune serum) contains antibodies to an organism. These do not stimulate an immune response, but simply provide immediate protection for an animal. They are usually used in the face of disease.

13. B *Dead vaccines are less long-lasting in effect than live vaccines*
Dead vaccines do not multiply within the animal so they only produce a relatively limited immune response. They require at least two injections for the initial vaccination course, and regular boosters to maintain the level of protection.
They are very safe because the organism is dead and cannot produce disease in its own right. However, because the immunity produced is not as good as for live vaccines, they are less widely used now than the live types.

14. B *Live attenuated vaccines should be stored between +2 and +8°C*

15. C *Mature antibody-producing cells are called B-cells*
These are a particular type of lymphocyte and they are
specific for a particular antigen. Monocytes pick up the
antigen and present it to B-cells until a correct match is found.
This causes the appropriate B-cell to multiply and start producing
antibodies against the antigen. The second type of lymphocyte,
the T-cell, is involved with cell-mediated immunity.

16. B *Animals are not routinely vaccinated before they reach 8–9*
weeks of age because there may still be maternal antibodies
within the plasma
After an animal is born it receives maternal antibodies from
colostrum, and these enter the neonate's bloodstream. These
antibodies can last within the circulation for up to 16 weeks, but
numbers gradually decline after about 4–6 weeks. If a vaccine
is given while there are still high levels of circulating maternal
antibodies the young animal has no need to produce its own
antibodies, since the maternal antibodies are available to act
against the antigen. However, after the maternal antibodies
have broken down there is no residual immunity. If the vaccine
is given once maternal antibody levels have decreased,
then the immune system of the pup or kitten is stimulated
to produce its own response, which has a much longer
lasting effect.

17. A *Monocytes are phagocytes*
Lymphocytes are not phagocytes, but are very important in the
immune response because one type (the B-cells) are capable
of producing antibodies, and the other type (T-cells) are
involved in the cell-mediated response.
The role of the basophil is not clearly understood, whereas
eosinophils are involved in allergic responses and parasitism.

18. B *An epidemic can be defined as a disease that has suddenly*
increased in prevalence in an area
A disease normally present within an area is described as
endemic. If there is a world-wide spread of a disease, it is
described as pandemic. If an epidemic of an animal disease
occurs, it can also be called an epizootic.

14 Elementary mycology and parasitology

1. C *An example of a pathogenic yeast is Candida*
Candida is sometimes found in chronic ear infections, and is the
organism responsible for sour crop in birds.
    Aspergillus, Trichophyton and Microsporum are all examples
of moulds.

2. B *The type of medium used to culture fungi is Sabouraud's
medium*
Selenite broth and deoxycholate citrate agar are both
selective media used to encourage the growth of Salmonella
bacteria. McConkey agar is another bacterial culture
medium used to identify lactose-fermenting bacteria
that can be grown in the presence of bile salts, such as
Escherichia coli.

3. B *The mite that can cause alopecia around the eyes and muzzle
without obvious pruritus is Demodex canis*
Otodectes cynotis is the ear mite which causes excessive
earwax production and intense irritation. Cheyletiella and
Sarcoptes mites both live on the body and produce pruritus.

4. C *The larval stage of Toxocara canis that is infective is the
second stage larvae (L_2)*
When eggs of Toxocara canis are passed in faeces, the
worm starts to develop within the egg. The first and
second stage larvae develop there, and it is when the
egg contains the L_2 larva that it is infective if ingested by
an animal.

5. A *The proper name of the hookworm is Uncinaria stenocephala*
There is also another hookworm occasionally seen in dogs
called Ancylostoma.
    Trichuris vulpis is the whipworm. Oslerus osleri is the canine
lungworm. This used to be called Filaroides osleri. Toxascaris
leonina is an intestinal roundworm similar in appearance to
Toxocara species.

6. B *Linognathus setosus is a sucking louse*
Sucking lice have mouthparts that enable them to suck blood
from their host. Linognathus is the sucking louse of the dog.

Trichodectes canis and Felicola subrostratus are both biting
lice that feed off the epidermis. Trichodectes is found in
the dog, and Felicola in the cat. There is no sucking louse of
the cat.

Ctenocephalides felis is the proper name for the
cat flea.

7. A *The larval form of Trombicula autumnalis is parasitic*
The nymph and adult forms of Trombicula are free-living, and
it is only the larvae that parasitize cats and dogs. The mites
are often found around the ears or feet, and can cause marked
irritation and self-excoriation.

Note, Trombicula can also be called Neotrombicula
autumnalis.

8. D *Taenia hydatigena always requires an intermediate host*
Taenia species are tapeworms, and all tapeworms require an
intermediate host because they have indirect life cycles.

Toxocara canis, Toxascaris leonina and Toxoplasma
gondii can all undergo direct life cycles, or may use
another host.

9. D *The parasite that typically causes intense pruritus and
crusting of the ear tips is Sarcoptes scabiei*
This is the way in which many Sarcoptes infestations first
appear clinically, but the mites quickly spread over the body
and the animal rapidly becomes covered in sores as it scratches
and bites at itself.

Demodex infestations are usually non-pruritic, unless there is
secondary bacterial infection. Trichodectes and Cheyletiella do
cause irritation, but can be found anywhere over the body.

10. A *Trichuris vulpis has distinctive lemon-shaped eggs with a plug
at each end*
The eggs of Toxascaris and Toxocara are round, and quite
similar to each other, except that the surface of the Toxocara
egg is more pitted.

Uncinaria eggs are oval, and several cells may be seen within
the shell.

11. D *The eggs of Linognathus setosus are glued to the hair shafts of its host*
All lice produce eggs which they cement to the hairs of the host. The eggs are often referred to as 'nits'.

12. C *Dermatophyte test medium turns red if fungi are cultured on its surface*
Dermatophyte test medium (DTM) is a variant on Sabouraud's medium, which contains an indicator that changes colour when a certain sugar is metabolized. Fungi use this sugar preferentially, so the medium changes colour from orange to deep red if they are present. Bacteria can also grow on the medium but use a different sugar first, and so do not produce the colour change.

13. B *Toxoplasma is not passed from queen to kitten via milk*
Toxoplasma can be transmitted via contaminated food, sheep abortions or meat from an intermediate host.

14. C *The term that describes infestation by dipteran larvae is 'myiasis'*
Dipteran larvae, or maggots, cause what is usually called fly-strike in animals. Flies lay their eggs on areas of the skin or fur that is soiled with faeces, blood or urine, and when the eggs hatch the maggots start to eat the contaminated tissues and then continue to burrow their way into healthy tissues.
Mydriasis is the term for pupil dilation and miosis is the opposite, meaning pupil constriction.
Meiosis is the type of cell division seen in the development of the sperm and ova.

15. C *The whipworm of dogs is Trichuris vulpis*
Aelurostrongylus abstrusus is the lungworm of the cat. Oslerus osleri is the lungworm of the dog, and Uncinaria stenocephala is the hookworm.

16. A *Pruritus and excessive epidermal scaling can be caused by the non-burrowing mite Cheyletiella*
Cheyletiella infestations are often seen in young animals, and are sometimes referred to as 'walking dandruff' because of the large amount of epidermal scaling.
Notoedres and Sarcoptes are both burrowing mites, seen in the cat and dog respectively. These also produce significant irritation.
Otodectes cynotis is a non-burrowing mite, but lives solely within the ear canals, causing localized irritation and increased production of earwax.

17. B *Taenia hydatigena reproduces asexually*
All tapeworms are hermaphroditic; that is, they contain the sexual organs of both the male and female. Toxocara cati, Ixodes ricinus (the sheep tick) and Felicola subrostratus are all parasites that reproduce sexually.

18. A *Visceral larva migrans in man is caused by Toxocara canis*
Visceral larva migrans occurs when a human is accidentally infected by Toxocara larvae. Since man is not the normal host, the larvae undergo part of their life cycle and migrate through body tissues before becoming dormant. In most cases this migration does not produce significant clinical effects, but in a small number of cases problems such as liver pain or neurological signs develop. The occurrence of clinical disease depends on which tissues the larvae migrate through or where they finish their migration. In a tiny proportion of cases the larvae lodge in the retina and provoke a granulomatous reaction, which causes partial or even total blindness in the affected eye.

Toxoplasma can also affect humans, and is particularly dangerous for women exposed to the organism for the first time during pregnancy. In about 10% of cases, this can lead to damage to the foetus or even abortion.

Echinococcus granulosus is another potential zoonosis, and can produce large hydatid cysts in man in the same way as it does within its normal intermediate host, the sheep.

19. D *A paratenic host is a host that carries the immature parasite within its tissues. It has to be eaten by the final host for the parasite to complete its life cycle*
A host in which a parasite has to undergo part of its life cycle before it can reinfest the final host is an intermediate host.

A host that carries an organism and sheds it intermittently is a transport host.

An animal in which the adult or reproductive phase of the parasite's life occurs is called the final or definitive host.

20. C *Wood's lamp examination will cause some Microsporum species to fluoresce*
Approximately 60% of Microsporum species will fluoresce when viewed using an ultra-violet light. The fungus shows as an apple-green fluorescence, usually most obvious at the edge of a lesion. However, starch and other substances can produce false positives, and some species do not fluoresce, so Wood's lamp results should be interpreted with caution. If the lesion is suspicious, then cultures should be made of hair plucks from the edge of the area for confirmation of the diagnosis.

21. B *The stain used to examine fungi is lactophenol cotton blue*
Gram's stain is used for bacterial identification. Wright's stain
is a Romanowsky stain that can be used for differential white
blood cell counts, and iodine is used either as part of Gram's
stain, or on its own to show undigested starches within faecal
smears.

15 General nursing

1. A *A decubitus ulcer is a pressure sore*
Decubitus ulcers are common complications in recumbent patients. They occur mainly over bony prominences, where the tissues are deprived of oxygen because the animal's weight compresses the blood vessels supplying the area.

2. C *Higginson's syringe can be used for giving an enema*
Higginson's syringe is a rubber pump that is used to transfer fluid from a container, through a bulb that is squeezed, and out through a narrow nozzle that is inserted into the animal's rectum.

   Sprawle's needle is a blunt-ended metal cannula used for irrigating the ear canal. A burette is used in combination with a giving set to deliver a specific volume via a drip. Fluid can be drawn from the thorax or abdomen simply by using a syringe and needle or syringe and catheter. When removing fluid from the thorax, it is helpful to use a three-way tap to ensure that air does not enter the pleural cavity. Alternatively, a mechanical chest drain can be used with a one-way valve.

3. B *Jackson's catheter should be used for catheterization of a cat*
Jackson's catheter is a short, fine, urinary catheter with a central wire stylet, which helps introduction of the catheter. It has a luer fitting, and a plastic collar with small holes in it so that it can be sutured to the skin and left as an indwelling catheter. Tieman's, Dowse's and Foley catheters are all used in the bitch.

4. B *If a patient had undergone oesophageal surgery, a gastrostomy tube would be the most appropriate method of forced feeding*
Oesophageal tissues do not heal very easily, and to avoid trauma to the area food should be given in such a way as to bypass the oesophagus. The best way is to use a gastrostomy tube. Liquid food can be administered via the tube, and the animal is sure to receive a balanced diet. Animals tolerate gastrostomy tubes well, and they can be placed at the time of surgery, either using an endoscope or a commercially available gastrostomy tube applicator.

5. B *You should suggest that they restrict protein in the diet and increase carbohydrate levels*

Protein should be restricted, as many older animals start to develop liver and kidney problems. These may not be clinically apparent, but by cutting down on surplus protein and changing the type of protein to something more readily digestible, it is possible to slow down the rate of deterioration of these organs. The carbohydrate levels require increasing simply to replace the calories that would previously have been supplied by protein.

Water should always be freely available. Acute renal failure can be precipitated by allowing animals to become dehydrated through inadequate fluid intake.

Energy levels should also be monitored closely. Most animals require fewer calories as they get older because their activity levels decrease.

Exercise is important for all animals, including older animals. However, this should be given little and often and on a regular basis to keep joints flexible, maintain the animal's interest, and provide ample opportunity for urination and defacation.

6. B *1 unit French Gauge is $\frac{1}{3}$ mm*

Catheters are measured in French Gauge (FG). This gives the external diameter of the catheter.

7. C *The disease that is not associated with older age is osteochondrosis*

Osteochondrosis is a disease seen in young animals, and usually presents clinically before the animal is a year old.

Periodontal disease and osteoarthritis are progressive conditions that usually start in middle to old age. Diabetes mellitus is also a disease that is classically seen in the middle-aged animal.

8. B *Dysphagia is difficulty eating*

9. B *The most serious complication of prolonged recumbency is hypostatic pneumonia*

If an animal is allowed to lie on one side for long periods of time, the lower lung becomes compressed by the animal's weight and is not aerated properly. Bronchial secretions also pool in the lower lung, and this provides an ideal medium in which bacteria can multiply. Turning a patient at least every

4 hours can help prevent this from occurring. Alternatively, propping a recumbent patient in sternal recumbency so that both lungs can be used will help. Coupage of the chest loosens bronchial secretions and enables the ciliated cells lining the respiratory tract to move the secretions up from the lungs.

Decubitus ulcers, joint stiffness and muscle wastage are all complications of prolonged recumbency, but are generally less life-threatening than hypostatic pneumonia. All can be avoided or minimized with good nursing care.

10. C *Constipation in patients can be prevented by the use of high fibre diets*
Fibre helps to prevent constipation by absorbing moisture and keeping the faeces fairly soft and easy for the animal to pass.

Kaolin is used to treat diarrhoea.

16 Medical disorders: infectious diseases

1. D *The cause of feline infectious anaemia is* Haemobartonella felis

Haemobartonella is a rickettsia that attaches itself onto the surface of red blood cells. Affected cells are destroyed as they pass through the spleen, giving rise to anaemia. The organism can be detected by making blood smears and staining them with Giemsa. The organism shows up as purple rings or cocci on the surface of the cells. Several blood samples may need to be taken over a period of time, as the organism is not always present within the circulation.

2. C *'Blue eye' is a complication encountered in dogs vaccinated with live canine adenovirus-1 vaccine*

'Blue eye' is so called because the cornea of the eye becomes opaque, which gives it a bluish sheen. It is caused by corneal oedema, the result of antigen–antibody complexes lodging within the cornea. It is seen in a very few cases, both in the naturally occurring disease and after vaccination with live attenuated canine adenovirus-1 (CAV-1). In most cases it resolves spontaneously, but in a tiny proportion of cases the pup is left with permanent scarring of the cornea.

To prevent this from occurring another vaccine is routinely used, which contains attenuated canine adenovirus-2 (CAV-2). This provides cross-protection for CAV-1, carries no risk of pups developing blue eye, and also protects against CAV-2, one of the organisms that produces respiratory disease as part of the kennel cough complex.

3. A *The cat should be isolated and retested in 3 months*

Over 40% of cats infected with feline leukaemia virus (FeLV) recover fully from the virus. These cats mount an immune response against the virus and throw off the infection without the development of FeLV-related diseases. Therefore, an apparently healthy cat should be isolated so that it is no risk to any other cats and then retested after about 12 weeks. If it is still carrying the virus, then it should be kept isolated and cared for until such time that it develops one of the FeLV-related diseases and its quality of life deteriorates. If the owner is unable to keep the cat isolated during this period, it is probably best that it is euthanased so that it does not present a risk to other healthy cats in the area.

4. B *The incubation period for parvovirus in dogs is 3–5 days*
Most viruses have quite short incubation periods. Leptospira
bacteria have a longer incubation period of between 7 and
21 days, and kennel cough has an incubation period of between
5 and 10 days.

5. C *Feline herpes virus 1 can become latent after an initial*
infection
After a primary infection, cats infected with feline herpes virus
apparently recover. However, the organism remains latent
(or hidden) within the body, where it is held in check by the
immune system. If the cat is stressed in some way, then the
herpes virus is able to multiply within tissues and clinical signs
redevelop. The main sign seen with herpes virus infection in
cats is upper respiratory tract disease.

6. D *Leptospira organisms may be found in both the blood and urine*
of infected animals
Animals with leptospirosis undergo bacteraemias in which the
bacteria circulate within the bloodstream and eventually
settle in either the liver, the kidney or both, depending on the
particular organism. They often remain within the interstitial
tissues of the kidney for many months after the clinical signs
of the disease regress, so urine from clinically recovered
animals can still contain viable bacteria. This is important with
regard to disease control.

7. B *Chlamydia infection in a cat can be diagnosed by microscopy of*
conjunctival scrapings
The scrapings are stained with Giemsa, and intracytoplasmic
inclusion bodies can be seen in affected cells.

8. B *A fomite is an inanimate object that becomes contaminated by a*
pathogenic organism and then comes into contact with a
non-infected animal
Organisms such as parvovirus, which are not easily destroyed
once out of the host, are often transferred between animals in
this way.

9. C *The fleas act as transport hosts for Haemobartonella felis*
Transport hosts are animals that carry a particular organism unchanged and are able to shed the organism at any time.

Biological vectors are hosts that are required by an organism for it to undergo part of its life cycle. Immature forms of the organism are found in the biological vector, and they are then passed on to a final host, where the adult or reproductive phase of the organism's life cycle occurs.

Intermediate hosts are the same thing, except that the term intermediate host is reserved for biological vectors that carry the immature stages of parasites.

10. C *Canine adenovirus-1 can cause acute pyrexia, petechial haemorrhages on the gums, hepatic enlargement, possible neurological signs, collapse and death in affected dogs*
Canine adenovirus-1 (CAV-1) causes the disease canine infectious hepatitis.

Acute myocarditis or gastro-enteritis is seen in parvovirus infections.

Canine distemper produces several different clinical syndromes, including respiratory signs, hyperkeratosis and neurological signs.

The group of organisms that form the kennel cough complex give rise to respiratory signs.

11. D *Leptospirosis is zoonotic*
Canine parvovirus, distemper virus and canine adenovirus-1 are all host-specific, and will not affect humans.

12. B *A saprophyte is an organism that lives on dead organic matter*
An organism that lives on a larger organism and causes disease is described as being pathogenic. Organisms that benefit their hosts are symbiotic or mutualistic, and organisms that do not have any effect on their hosts are described as commensals. However, if the immune system of the host is compromised, many commensals can become opportunist pathogens.

13. C *Viral diseases can be positively diagnosed in the live animal by checking for a rising antibody titre*
Paired blood samples are taken from the animal approximately 2 weeks apart, and antibody levels to the particular organism are measured. Animals that show an increase in

the antibody levels are actively mounting an immune response
against the infection, and are therefore definitely
carrying the virus.

14. C *The organism responsible for feline infectious peritonitis is not
resistant to many disinfectants, and does not remain in the
environment for very long.*
Feline infectious peritonitis (FIP) is caused by a coronavirus.
The virus is readily destroyed by most disinfectants,
and is easily killed by heat and drying. However, its mode of
transmission is not well understood; even apparently
isolated households can be affected by the disease, and the
incubation period is very variable. Two forms of FIP
are seen clinically: the wet form, in which a proteinaceous
fluid forms within body cavities; and the dry form, in
which micro-abscesses develop in the major organs of
the body.

15. C *Canine parvovirus is thought to have evolved from feline
panleucopenia virus*
Feline panleucopenia (also called feline infectious enteritis) is
caused by a parvovirus, which results in severe enteritis. The
canine parvovirus is very similar – so similar, in fact, that when
canine parvovirus infections were first seen, feline enteritis
vaccines were used in dogs to try and halt the spread of the
disease.

16. C *Feline calici virus causes chronic stomatitis and gingivitis*
Feline calici virus is one of the feline viruses that can cause
chronic infections in cats. Affected animals may continue to
shed the virus throughout their life, and often redevelop
clinical signs. The intracellular organism Chlamydia
psittaci also produces chronic disease, though the signs
associated with this tend to be ocular discharges and
conjunctivitis.

17. A *Canine parvovirus can last in the environment for up
to a year*
The parvoviruses are very resistant to many disinfectants, heat
and desiccation, and can therefore remain viable within the
environment for long periods of time.

18. B *Isolated cases should always be treated after the remainder of the inpatients*

Potentially infectious or contaminated animals should always be handled and treated last, so that the risk of disease transmission from these animals to those without infections is minimized. Ideally, infectious patients should be looked after by someone different from the person dealing with the rest of the animals, but this is not always possible. Protective clothing should always be worn, and nursing staff should disinfect themselves going into and out of an isolation ward. Isolation areas should have their own sets of food bowls, bedding and cleaning materials, so that nothing has to come out of the isolation area.

19. D *A neonate exposed to the feline leukaemia virus is most likely to become persistently infected with the virus*

Cats exposed to feline leukaemia virus (FeLV) before the immune system has had a chance to develop have the highest chance of becoming persistently infected and suffering from the FeLV-related diseases. Cats over 4 months of age have a much better survival rate after exposure, and up to 40% of these animals will recover from infection without long-term problems.

Kittens born from vaccinated cats, which have therefore received maternal antibodies via colostrum, are less at risk than those born to unvaccinated queens.

17 Medical disorders: non-infectious diseases

1. D *Diets containing restricted levels of protein and sodium should be given to animals with renal failure*

Protein should be restricted to avoid the build-up of toxic metabolites such as urea, which cannot be cleared quickly from the body by the diseased kidneys. Sodium should also be restricted to prevent fluid retention and the development of hypertension.

High fibre diets can be used in the management of animals with colitis. Food allergies should be treated using very simple diets that contain nutrient sources the animal has not encountered before.

Cats with feline urologic syndrome (FUS) require diets that have restricted mineral contents, and that result in the production of urine which has a pH that does not encourage the development of uroliths.

2. A *A hyperthyroid cat would not show bradycardia*

Hyperthyroid animals produce excessive amounts of the thyroid hormones T_3 and T_4. These hormones drive the animal's metabolism, and in excess result in very high metabolic rates. The clinical signs of weight loss, polyphagia, heat intolerance, mild diarrhoea and tachycardia are the result of the metabolic changes.

3. D *The cardiac disease that is congenital is persistent right aortic arch*

Persistent right aortic arch arises because the aorta develops from the right aortic arch rather than the left. As a result, the oesophagus becomes trapped between the aorta, the ligamentum arteriosum and the pulmonary vein. The circulatory system functions perfectly normally, but clinical signs are seen because food does not pass through the narrowed oesophagus easily, and so the animal starts to regurgitate food and a megaoesophagus develops cranial to the stricture. The ligamentum arteriosum can be transected surgically but it may be too late for the oesophagus to return to normal, in which case the animal will need to be fed semi-liquid food from a height so that gravity helps it slide down into the stomach.

Endocardiosis is seen mainly in older animals. Nodules develop on the valvular flaps and prevent them from closing properly. The condition worsens gradually, and may eventually lead to the development of heart failure.

Cardiomyopathies can arise either as primary conditions or secondary to other diseases, such as hyperthyroidism in cats. The heart muscle is affected so that it no longer functions adequately to maintain cardiac output.

Myocarditis is inflammation of the cardiac muscle. This usually develops as the result of some type of infection, for example parvovirus in very young pups. It is quite rare.

4. A *The clinical sign not typically associated with small intestinal diarrhoea is tenesmus*
Tenesmus, or straining, is most commonly seen with large intestinal problems.

In small intestinal diarrhoea weight loss is common because the animal is not able to digest or absorb its food normally, and as a result of this it is usually ravenously hungry. Borborygmi or increased gut sounds are also common.

5. D *Keto-acidosis can develop as a complication of diabetes mellitus*
In diabetes mellitus there is an absence of the insulin needed to drive glucose into cells. The cells therefore have to use an alternative energy source, and will use fatty acids and glycerol instead. Metabolism of these molecules leads to the formation of acidic ketone compounds as by-products. These accumulate within the circulation and can lead to life-threatening acidosis.

6. C *An animal suffering from left-sided heart failure would show pulmonary oedema leading to a cough*
In left-sided heart failure the left ventricle is not able to push sufficient blood into the systemic circulation to meet the body's demands. A 'back-log' of blood develops in the left atrium, and dams back into the pulmonary circulation. As pressure in the pulmonary vessels increases, fluid is pushed out of the capillaries into the alveolar spaces, and pulmonary oedema develops.

In right-sided failure a similar situation arises, except that the blood accumulates within the systemic circulation so that the major veins become distended and central venous pressure increases. This can cause a jugular pulse and the development of ascites and oedema. The heart muscle hypertrophies in response to cardiac failure. The right side enlarges in right-sided failure, and the left increases in left-sided failure.

7. **A** *Furunculosis is a severe example of pyoderma*
Furunculosis is a very deep skin infection, often caused by anaerobic bacteria. The most common sites for it to develop are around the anus, especially in German Shepherds with low tail carriage, and in the feet.

8. **C** *Orthopneoea is used to describe the case where the animal assumes sternal recumbency and breathes through its mouth*
This is seen when animals are in severe respiratory distress. Generally they find it impossible to lie down on their side, since this further compromises the function of the lower lung.

9. **C** *Salt should be decreased in patients with cardiac disease*
Reducing salt levels decreases water retention by the body, and therefore helps to lower blood pressure. Reducing the circulating blood volume decreases the workload on the heart, and prevents rapid deterioration of the patient's condition.

10. **D** *Jaundice can be caused by increased red blood cell destruction, bile duct obstruction or liver disease*
Jaundice develops when there is excess bilirubin within the circulation. Bilirubin is produced as a waste product of haemoglobin breakdown, and is normally processed by the liver and excreted via bile into the intestine.
    If any of these processes are affected by disease, there can be an increase in bilirubin levels resulting in jaundice.

11. **D** *Arterial blood pressure is at its maximum during ventricular systole*
The term systole is used to describe cardiac muscle contraction, and diastole describes relaxation of the muscle. The period during which arterial pressure is at its maximum is when the ventricles are actively contracting and pushing the blood into the arteries, which is ventricular systole.

12. **B** *Isosthenuria means that the kidney is unable either to dilute or concentrate urine, so produces urine similar in composition to protein-free plasma*

13. B *The bone condition associated with chronic renal failure is*
rubber jaw
In renal failure, phosphate is retained within the circulation. The
calcium–phosphorus balance is therefore upset, and parathyroid
hormone (PTH) is released to increase blood calcium levels to
restore the balance again. PTH stimulates bone resorption, so
bones eventually become weakened and soft. This is
particularly noticeable in the jaw. If the mandibles of
anaesthetized patients with this condition are squeezed gently,
there is abnormal bending of the bones. This is painful if tried
in the conscious animal.

Marie's disease is a condition in which there is bone
proliferation on the distal long bones, causing pain and
lameness. This occurs in response to the presence of
intrathoracic masses, although it is not well understood why.

Lion jaw is another proliferative bone disease. The mandibles
of affected animals are inflamed, and it is painful for the
animal to open and close its mouth. There may be new bone
laid down around the temporo-mandibular joint, which restricts
the range of movement of the joint. It is most commonly seen
in West Highland White Terriers. The cause is not understood,
but in most cases progression of the disease stops once the
animal reaches skeletal maturity.

Barlow's disease or metaphyseal osteopathy is another
disease with no clear cause. The metaphyses (the areas adjacent
to the growth plates) are enlarged, and are hot and painful for
the animal. Damage can extend to the growth plate and cause
limb deformities, but in most cases the condition resolves
completely as the animal gets older.

14. B *Foods allergies can be diagnosed using restriction diets*
Animals with suspect food allergies should initially be kept on
very simple diets containing foods that they have not
encountered before. If the allergy signs improve, then new
foods can be added, one at a time, until the symptoms return
and the problem food identified. Intradermal testing can be
used to identify contact or inhaled allergens.

Antihistamines will mask the clinical effects of allergies,
regardless of the cause, and so are of no use in diagnosis, although
they are widely used in the management of allergies and atopies.

15. D *The hormones responsible for calcium regulation are*
parathyroid hormone and calcitonin
The thyroid hormones control metabolic rate.

Glucocorticoids are released in response to stress to keep blood glucose levels high. Mineralocorticoids are needed to maintain sodium and potassium balance within the body. Insulin and glucagon are responsible for the regulation of blood glucose levels.

16. **B** *Pentobarbitone can be used in the management of a fitting animal*
In cases of status epilepticus, pentobarbitone (Sagatal) is often used to induce a long-lasting anaesthesia. The brain's activity is suppressed, and the hope is that once the effects of the anaesthetic wear off, the focus of the epileptic fit will remain quiet.
Phenyl propanolamine (Propalin) is used in the treatment of urinary incontinence.
Prednisolone is a short-acting glucocorticoid that can be used to treat inflammatory or auto-immune conditions.
Phenylbutazone is a non-steroidal anti-inflammatory widely used in the management of osteoarthritis.

17. **D** *The hormone released by the kidney when blood pressure falls is renin*
Renin is released as soon as glomerular perfusion decreases. It stimulates the conversion of inactive angiotensinogen in the circulation into the active form, angiotensin. Angiotensin causes vasoconstriction, and so increases blood pressure, and also stimulates the adrenal cortex to release the hormone aldosterone. Aldosterone encourages sodium retention, so that water is also retained and blood pressure is further increased.
Erythropoietin is also produced by the kidney, but is produced continuously. It acts on the bone marrow to stimulate the maturation of red blood cells.

18. **C** *Endocardiosis causes the development of nodules on the cusps of the heart valves, which prevents them opening and closing normally, and is the most common cause of congestive heart failure in the dog*
This is common, especially in certain breeds such as the Cavalier King Charles Spaniel. Clinical signs start to show as the animal reaches middle age, and worsen with age.
Pericardial effusions result from several different conditions, including infections or tumours. Fluid accumulates within the pericardial cavity causing compression of the heart, especially

the weaker right side. The heart can no longer pump efficiently, and signs of heart failure develop.

Endocarditis is the result of blood-borne infections reaching the endothelium of the heart, causing inflammation and disease. Animals are normally pyrexic and lethargic. Long courses of systemic antibiotics are needed to treat these cases.

Myocarditis is inflammation of heart muscle, again usually caused by infection. This is quite rare now, although it used to be seen in very young pups with acute parvovirus infections.

19. D *Increased serum amylase and lipase activities usually suggest pancreatic disease*
Inflammation of the pancreas causes release of the digestive enzymes amylase and lipase into the circulation. These are not normally present in the bloodstream.

18 Obstetrics and paediatrics

1. B *Oestrus can be prevented, suppressed or postponed by using progestagens*
Progestagens are drugs that mimic the effect of progesterone. Progesterone is produced during pregnancy by the corpus luteum, and acts to keep the uterus in the state needed to maintain the pregnancy. It also acts on the anterior pituitary to prevent the release of follicle stimulating hormone (FSH) and luteinizing hormone (LH). In the absence of FSH and LH the animal will not come into heat, and therefore will not ovulate. Using progestagens has the same effect.

2. B *The post-parturient condition that causes shivering, muscle spasm, collapse and disorientation in the lactating bitch is lactation tetani (eclampsia)*
Lactation tetani or eclampsia is caused by low blood calcium. The bitch produces so much milk that her readily available supplies of calcium are used up, and her blood levels fall. This results in failure of normal nerve and muscle function. Without rapid calcium supplementation the bitch could die, so these cases must be considered as medical emergencies. Intravenous calcium borogluconate should be given until the clinical signs start to resolve.
   Metritis is inflammation of the uterus, usually caused by bacteria entering the uterus through the cervix during parturition. Mastitis is inflammation and infection of the mammary glands. Parvovirus infection in the adult animal causes severe vomiting and diarrhoea. However, if the bitch had been vaccinated it would not produce significant disease.

3. B *Neonates will not receive the full value of colostrum if it is given later than 36 hours after birth, because they are unable to absorb the antibodies directly into the bloodstream*
If an animal drinks colostrum shortly after birth, the antibodies in the colostrum are not digested as normal proteins would be but are absorbed directly into the intestinal capillaries. These antibodies provide protection for the neonate against diseases that the mother has either been exposed to or vaccinated against.
   After 24–36 hours, the intestinal wall in the young animal changes and the antibodies are no longer absorbed unchanged but are digested in the same way as other proteins. The change in the intestinal wall is known as closure, and it is one of the

main reasons that it is imperative for a neonate to receive an adequate supply of colostrum in the first few hours after birth.

4. C *Pups' and kittens' eyes open 10–14 days after birth*

5. D *None of the statements are true*
The queen is a seasonal breeder, which means that there are only certain times of the year that she will come into season. The season starts in the spring and continues through to the autumn. She is polyoestrous, which means that during this time she will show several oestrous cycles before entering anoestrus.
   The queen is an induced ovulator, so she will only ovulate once she has been mated. A queen that is not mated will therefore enter oestrus several times during a breeding season, but will not actually ovulate.

6. C *Uterine inertia is not a type of foetal dystocia*
Dystocias can be classified as maternal or foetal, depending on the cause. Foetal dystocias arise due to foetal oversize, an abnormal foetus or some type of malpresentation. Maternal dystocias include uterine inertia, birth canal abnormalities or some other physical obstruction.

7. B *The puerperium is the term used to describe the period after birth during which the uterus returns to normal*
The uterus usually takes between 4 and 6 weeks to involute or return to its normal size.

8. C *The hormone present through metoestrus in the bitch is progesterone*
Follicle stimulating hormone (FSH) is produced during proestrus, and is the hormone that causes follicular maturation. As the follicles mature they release oestrogen, which increases in concentration until it peaks just prior to ovulation. The peak in oestrogen levels triggers a surge in luteinizing hormone (LH), which stimulates ovulation and the development of the corpus luteum. The LH surge occurs during oestrus.
   The corpus luteum produces progesterone for several weeks after ovulation. This phase is metoestrus, after which the corpus luteum regresses and the bitch, if not pregnant, returns to anoestrus.

9. D *No drugs can be used in the event of a misalliance in the queen*
In the bitch, oestrogen compounds such as oestrodiol benzoate can be used to terminate a misalliance and bring the animal

back into oestrus, providing they are given within 4 days of mating.

Oestrogens cannot be used in the queen, as they are relatively toxic to cats and cause bone marrow suppression. The only options are either to allow the pregnancy to continue or to spay the cat.

10. **D** *The average duration of oestrus in the bitch is 9 days*
The average timings for the stages of the oestrus cycle in the bitch are: proestrus 9 days; oestrus 9 days; metoestrus 50–60 days; anoestrus 4 months.

This gives a total oestrous cycle of 7 months. However, these are only average figures, and individual animals can show wide variations from these timings.

11. **D** *A breech birth occurs when a foetus is delivered in posterior longitudinal presentation, dorsal position with hindlimbs flexed*
The terms 'presentation', 'position' and 'posture' can be used to define accurately the way a pup or kitten is delivered. A breech birth occurs when the pup is coming backwards and the right way up, but the legs are flexed so that it is trying to come out bottom first. Often these pups cannot be delivered easily, and assistance is required.

12. **C** *If an animal is primigravid, it means that this is her first litter*
The term multigravid refers to an animal that has had one or more litters previously.

Uniparous describes a species that normally only carries one foetus.

13. **B** *A week-old orphan pup being hand reared should be fed every 4 hours*
Up to 1 week of age it should be fed every 2 hours, but this can be decreased to every 4 hours at a week of age, providing the pup is growing well and putting on weight. Over the next 2 weeks the frequency of feeding can gradually be reduced to just 4 feeds a day. Once the pup reaches 3 weeks of age, it is possible to start introducing solid foods as well as milk feeds.

14. **D** *Progesterone is tested for to determine whether a bitch is ready for mating or not*
Progesterone is only produced after ovulation has occurred and the corpus luteum has formed, and so it is the only reliable

indicator of ovulation. The other hormones are present before and during oestrus, and so do not provide any indication of when to mate the bitch. If a bitch is mated within 2 days of ovulating, the chances of conception are good.

15. D *If a vaginal smear taken was taken from a bitch during oestrus, the predominant cells would be cornified cells*
An alternative method to blood testing is to use vaginal smears to determine when a bitch comes into oestrus.

In proestrus, the main cell types are red blood cells and some round epithelial cells. As the bitch moves towards oestrus, the red blood cells decrease in number, and the epithelial cells becomes more crenated and do not have nuclei.

Smears taken in metoestrus show the presence of many white blood cells.

16. B *Strabismus is a squint*
This is seen as a normal finding in many kittens, and in most cases it resolves as they get older. However, many Siamese retain the squint throughout their lives.

17. A *Semen for artificial insemination (AI) is usually collected from the tom cat using electro-ejaculation*
In the dog, the most usual methods are either digital manipulation or the use of an artificial vagina.

18. D *Vaginal smears can be stained using Leishman's, Wright's or Difquik stains*
Any of the Romanowsky stains can be used for staining vaginal smears. Romanowsky stains contain two dyes; a blue dye that stains alkaline areas, and a red dye that has an affinity for acidic areas within cells. In this way, different types of cells can be readily identified.

19. C *The ferret is an induced ovulator*
As well as the cat, the ferret and the rabbit are induced ovulators. Most other small animal species are spontaneous ovulators.

20. B *Palpation can be used as a method of pregnancy diagnosis after 3–4 weeks of the pregnancy*
At this stage, the foetuses are just detectable as small swellings within the uterus. Individual parts of the foetuses cannot be distinguished until they are about 6–7 weeks old.

It is not possible to tell the number of foetuses accurately through palpation.

21. C *The foetal membranes are passed during the third stage of parturition*
Parturition is classically divided into three stages. The first stage is the preparation phase. The pregnant animal starts nesting, and is restless and unsettled. She may show intermittent contractions.

During the second stage, the female undergoes regular uterine contractions and gives birth to the offspring. This is followed by the third stage, when the foetal membranes are passed. In animals giving birth to several young, the second and third stages may occur together with each foetus being followed by its membranes, or a few young may be born and then the membranes follow later.

There is no fourth stage of parturition.

22. C *A whelping kennel should be maintained at 26°C*
This is to ensure that the pups do not become hypothermic during their first days of life, since they are unable to thermoregulate at this age. If the pups are orphaned or have to be kept on their own initially, then the temperature should be even higher (up to 30°C). This can gradually be reduced over a 2-week period as the pups develop.

23. C *The term used for a developing pup once it is approximately 35 days old and has recognizable features is a foetus*
The fertilized egg is called a zygote or conceptus until implantation occurs. From this time until it becomes a foetus, the developing pup is called an embryo.

19 General surgical nursing

1. D *Paracentesis is not a laparotomy approach*
Paracentesis is the removal of fluid from the abdomen via a
needle or catheter.

The pararectal approach describes an incision made parallel but
to one side of the midline, parallel to the rectus abdominis muscle.

The paracostal approach is made parallel to the costal arch,
following the line of the last rib.

The sublumbar or flank approach is the laparotomy approach
most frequently used for cat speys.

2. D *The Ehmer sling can be used after luxation and replacement of
the hip joint*
If the shoulder joint is dislocated, then a Velpeau sling can be
used after its replacement.

Robert–Jones bandages could be used if support was needed
after treatment of stifle or elbow dislocations.

3. D *Plaster of Paris takes over 12 hours to reach full
weight-bearing strength*
Plaster of Paris may set quite quickly, but it does not reach full
weight-bearing strength until it is completely dry. This can take
over 24 hours.

Newer casting materials are now frequently used to overcome
this problem, and most are strong as soon as they are
cool – often within 30 minutes.

4. C *A gastropexy might be indicated in the management of a
gastric torsion*
In a gastric torsion the stomach twists about the oesophagus,
which prevents the stomach contents from exiting normally into
the intestine. The gastric secretions continue to be produced, and
the stomach becomes progressively enlarged with fluid and gas.
This causes compression of the vena cava, which compromises
venous return to the heart. The blood supply to the stomach wall
is also affected, since the vessels are trapped in the twist. Without
rapid treatment animals with gastric torsions will die, and even
those that do receive treatment may die later due to the effect of
toxins released into the bloodstream when the stomach is
returned to its normal position.

To prevent a torsion recurring a gastropexy can be performed,
in which the stomach is sutured to the body wall to fix it in
position.

5. A *A wedge biopsy would provide the most information about a lump that was suspected of being a tumour*
If a small 'pie slice' of a lump is taken, fixed in formalin solution, and sent for histopathology, thin slices can be prepared for examination. Since the sample submitted contains cells from the edge and the centre of the lump, the sample should be truly representative of the whole lesion. An accurate diagnosis should then be possible.

A needle biopsy can be used in situations where it is not possible to remove the whole mass. However, the sample taken is much smaller than a wedge biopsy, and there is a chance that the cells collected may not be typical of the cell types present.

Needle aspirates are less accurate still, as literally only a few cells are collected and squirted out onto a slide so that a smear can be made. This technique is most often used in the diagnosis of lymphosarcoma, where the presence of abnormal lymphocytes can be diagnostic.

Exfoliative cytology is really only of use in situations where none of the other techniques are feasible. In this method, cells are collected from the surface of the suspected tumour. For nasal or prostatic examinations, a solution of sterile saline is flushed back and forth over the area and then collected. It is then spun down and the sediment examined. It is quite common to get non-diagnostic samples using this method.

6. C *Intra-ocular pressure is not decreased in glaucoma*
In glaucoma, there is an increase in intra-ocular pressure due to lack of drainage of the aqueous humour in the anterior compartment of the eye. It can be caused either by trauma or through an inherited condition. Left untreated, the pressure within the globe increases to the degree that the retina is damaged and the animal starts to lose vision in the affected eye.

7. D *The Yorkshire Terrier shows an increased incidence of tracheal collapse*

8. C *Urethral calculi could be an indication for performing a urethrostomy in a male animal*
Urethral calculi can often lodge in the narrow urethra of the male animal. In the cat, this usually occurs in the terminal urethra close to the penis. In the dog, the calculi often lodge at the base of the os penis. It may be possible to flush the

calculi back into the bladder when this occurs, but if it has been a recurrent problem it may be better to create a permanent urethrostomy above the point at which the calculi lodge. Diet modifications should also be made to try and prevent the formation of the calculi.

Ruptured bladder, ectopic ureters and hydronephrosis all require surgical management. Hydronephrosis usually requires a nephrectomy of the affected kidney and removal of the ureter. Ectopic ureters can be implanted into the trigone of the bladder, and a ruptured bladder should be surgically repaired.

9. A *Orchidectomy is the surgical removal of one or both testes*
Removal of a section of the vas deferens is termed a vasectomy. This is rarely performed in cats and dogs, but can be carried out in ferrets because the female (jill) has to be mated in order to come out of oestrus.

Penile amputations are unusual, but indications could include severe trauma, or a perineal urethrostomy in a tom cat.

10. B *A transverse fracture of a long bone could be repaired using a plate*
A transverse fracture of a long bone is an unstable fracture, where there tends to be rotation of the fragments relative to each other unless they are fixed in some way. Casts, intramedullary pins and splints will prevent most types of movement at the fracture site, but do nothing to provide rotational stability. A bone plate is the only repair device that provides sufficient immobilization of the fracture fragments to allow the bone to heal.

11. A *Animals with lymphosarcoma are most commonly treated using chemotherapy*
Several cytotoxic drugs have been used in the management of lymphosarcoma. These include vincristine (Oncovin), cyclophosphamide (Endoxana) and prednisolone. It is important during treatment that the patient's red and white blood cell counts are monitored, since the drugs are toxic to all dividing cells and not just cancerous cells, and bone marrow suppression is a potential side effect.

Surgery, and complete excision of tumours, is the management of choice for single growths, but is not always possible. Radiotherapy can be used for some tumours that are difficult to operate on. These need to be reasonably superficial, such as oral or nasal tumours, to achieve adequate penetration of the tumour by radiation. Radioactive isotopes are used only rarely, since the patients need to be hospitalized somewhere with adequate radiation protection facilities. Isotopes are sometimes used in the management of thyroid tumours, using radioactive iodine.

12. C *Fracture disease is the term used to describe the situation which arises when scar formation after fracture healing has occurred and prevents normal limb usage*
Infection of the bone and bone marrow is osteomyelitis. This is often caused by poor aseptic technique during surgery.
   Malunion occurs when the bone heals but the alignment is abnormal.
   When implants such as plates and screws are being used, it is essential that they are made of the same metal. If they are not, an electric current is set up between them and the bone becomes damaged by electrolysis. Eventually the implants loosen and fall out, and bone healing will not occur.

13. C *The first thing that should be tried when dealing with a suspect gastric torsion is to pass a stomach tube*
If passing a stomach tube is successful, it will allow gas and fluid to be released from the stomach. This will decrease the pressure on the vena cava and on the gastric wall, and slow the development of severe shock. It is a non-invasive technique that could save the animal's life.
   If this does not work, then the next thing to do is to trocharize the abdomen using a large-gauge needle. This should only be carried out under a veterinary surgeon's direction. This also reduces the pressure on the vena cava and provides more time to prepare for other procedures such as surgery.

14. C *An osteochondroma is a benign tumour*
Tumours that have names ending in -sarcoma or -carcinoma are malignant tumours. A malignant melanoma should strictly be called a melanocarcinoma. Most melanomas in small animals are malignant.

15. C *Cyanosis is not a cardinal sign of inflammation*
There are five basic signs of inflammation, which together are referred to as the 'cardinal signs'. These are redness, swelling, pain, heat and loss of function.

16. B *The lens is affected by the development of cataracts*
Cataracts are opacities that develop on or within the lens. Some
cataracts can be removed and the lens left intact;
others can only be treated by surgical removal of the lens
(lentectomy).

17. D *Gangrene is the death of tissues, with or without bacterial
invasion*

18. A *If an animal is suffering from keratitis, the cornea is inflamed*
Inflammation of the conjunctiva is called conjunctivitis, and
blepharitis is the term used when the eyelids are inflamed. If
the sclera becomes inflamed, then it is described as scleritis or
episcleritis.

19. B *Rush pins are often used in pairs in the repair of epiphyseal
fractures*
Rush pins are small bone pins with a hook at one end and a
sledge runner tip at the other. They are placed obliquely so that
the sledge runner tip contacts, but does not pass through, the
opposite cortex of the bone. They are useful for epiphyseal
fractures because they cause minimum disruption to the growth
plate and the bone can therefore continue to grow as well as
heal.
  A Steinmann pin is a large intramedullary pin frequently
used in orthopaedic surgery. This would not be suitable for the
repair of this type of fracture, as it is unlikely that the pin would
have sufficient hold on the small epiphyseal fragment.
  A Kuntscher nail is another type of intramedullary pin. It has
either a V- or clover-shaped cross-section, which gives a better
hold than the Steinmann pin within the medullary cavity.

20. B *A drain could be used for a deep wound in which dead space
has been created by the surgical removal of some tissue*
A drain is a device that allows air to enter and fluid to flow
from deep tissues to the surface. Drains are often used after
tissue removal to allow serum to drain from the area and
prevent it accumulating within the dead space.

20 Theatre practice and care and maintenance of surgical instruments

1. **B** *Scrubbed personnel should pass each other back to back*
   Passing back to back minimizes the risk of contaminating the most important sterile area, the front of the person. It is also important that a scrubbed person does not turn his or her back to the operating table.

2. **B** *The area should not be prepared centripetally working in towards the site of the incision*
   When a surgical site is prepared, the scrub solution should always be applied working outwards from the site of the skin incision, and never back towards the centre.
   Before starting the surgical scrub, it is always important to ensure that as much gross contamination and hair has been removed from the site as possible.

3. **A** *Sterilization cannot be achieved by boiling*
   Boiling will produce disinfection but not sterilization, as it will not kill bacterial spores. Autoclaving, infra-red radiation and ethylene oxide can all be used to sterilize equipment.

4. **C** *Drapes should be placed closest to the person spreading the drapes first, then on the opposite side, followed by the two ends*
   The drape closest is placed first so that the sterile person placing the drapes does not risk contamination by leaning across and touching the patient. The drape on the opposite side can then be placed so that the surgeon or second scrubbed person can come close to the patient safely. Finally the two end drapes are placed, and all are held in place with towel clips.

5. **B** *Hot air ovens do not require lower temperatures than autoclaves*
   Operating temperatures for hot air ovens are between 150°C and 180°C, depending on the substance being sterilized. The temperatures for autoclaves are between 121°C and 134°C, depending on the pressure generated.
   Instruments being sterilized by hot air ovens are laid out on perforated trays ready for use. The hot air should be able to circulate freely around the instruments, therefore the oven should not be overloaded. Sharp instruments start to blunt with

repeated heating and should be sterilized using the coolest temperature (150°C) for 180 minutes. Since no moisture is used in this technique, petroleum jelly, powders and other chemicals can be sterilized by hot air ovens.

6. B *An operating theatre should not have two entrances*
A theatre should only have one entrance, so that it is not a thoroughfare to any other room and only the minimum number of people are present during an operating session. The theatre should be for surgical procedures only, with all preparation of the patient, surgeon, and assistants carried out in a separate preparation area.

It is very helpful to have X-ray viewing facilities in theatre.

7. C *The holding time for sterilizing instruments in an autoclave operating at a pressure of 15 lb/sq. in (1.2 kg/cm^2) and a temperature of 121°C is 15 minutes*

8. B *Gamma radiation is used to sterilize surgical gloves*
Gamma radiation is used for most disposables, including surgical gloves, suture materials, catheters and needles. Infra-red radiation is used for syringes.

9. B *A cystotomy would be classified as a clean-contaminated operation*
A clean operation is one in which there is no break in asepsis, and none of the uro-genital, respiratory or gastro-intestinal tracts are entered.

A clean–contaminated operation is one in which a contaminated area is entered, but there is no spillage of the contents. This constitutes a minor break in asepsis.

A contaminated operation is when there a leakage from the gastro-intestinal or uro-genital tracts, or marked inflammation. There is, however, no infection present. Contaminated surgery includes the management of open, fresh traumatic wounds.

A dirty operation is one in which there is pus and infection present.

10. D *The sterility monitor that responds to temperature and time only is Browne's tube*
Browne's tubes can be used in either an autoclave or hot air oven, providing the correct tube is chosen. After the specified temperature and time is reached, the liquid inside the tube changes from red to green.

Sterigauge and TST strips respond to temperature, steam and time, and so are useful for monitoring autoclave efficiency.

Autoclave tape only shows that steam has penetrated the area where the tape was positioned. It does not give any indication that the correct temperature was reached, or that the steam was present for the appropriate amount of time. This is the least reliable method of testing for sterility.

11. D *The suture material that remains the longest within a wound before it is broken down by enzymes is polydioxanone (PDS)*
Polydioxanone loses half its strength in 50 days, but is not totally absorbed until after 180 days. Polyglactin 910 (Vicryl) and Polyglycolic acid (Dexon) are totally absorbed after about 100 days. Catgut is the suture material that lasts the shortest time. Plain catgut is totally broken down in 15 days, whereas chromic catgut, which is more commonly used, lasts for 30 days.

The way in which absorbable suture materials are removed from wounds depends from what they are made. Natural suture materials (such as catgut) are removed by phagocytosis, whereas synthetic sutures are removed by enzymes that cause hydrolysis.

12. C *Assuming no complications, skin sutures should usually be removed 7–10 days after surgery*
Under good healing conditions, most surgical skin wounds heal after about 5–7 days. The recommendation of removal after 7–10 days therefore allows a few extra days to make sure the tissue is strong enough.

This would not necessarily be long enough in all situations. If there had been tension on the sutures, contamination by bacteria, or animal interference with the wound, then the sutures might need to be left in place for longer.

13. A *In old nomenclature, 2/0 suture material is one size thicker than 3/0*
The BPC gauges start with 10/0 as the finest material, and increase in size to 2/0. 0 is the next size up, and the sizes then increase from 1 to 6.

The metric system is more logical. The number of the suture gives the diameter of the thread in mm multiplied by 10. Therefore, 5 metric has a diameter of 0.5 mm.

There is no easy way to convert between the two systems, but two of the more commonly used sizes are 2/0, which is the equivalent of 3 metric, and 3/0, which is the same as 2 metric.

14. B *The horizontal mattress suture is an everting pattern*
This means that the wound edges have a tendency to pucker up, and do not lie flat.

The other suture patterns – simple interrupted, cruciate mattress and Ford interlocking – all produce good wound edge apposition, with no inversion or eversion.

15. A *0.2 metric is the smallest suture material size available*
In BPC gauge this is the same as 10/0.

16. C *The suture material that is monofilament is polypropylene (Prolene)*
Silk, catgut and Polyglactin 910 (Vicryl) are all braided suture materials.

17. A *A curved cutting needle would appear triangular in cross section, with the apex of the triangle on the inside of the curve*
The reverse cutting needle is similar, except that the apex is on the outside of the curve. Cutting needles are usually used for skin and tough tissues.

The needle with a round cross-section and fine tapered point is described as round bodied, and is relatively atraumatic.

18. A *Wire suture material is sized in Gauge, e.g. 20 G*
The numbers decrease as the wire gets thicker, so the coarsest is 18 G and the finest is 40 G.

19. A *The retractor that is not self-retaining is the Langenbek retractor*
The Langenbek retractor is a hand-held retractor, whereas the Travers, Gossett and Gelpi retractors are all self-retaining.

20. D *Cortical screws are more tightly threaded than cancellous screws*
Cortical screws are designed for use in dense cortical bone. The shaft is wider than the shaft in cancellous screws of the same diameter, and the thread is tighter. Cortical screws are usually fully threaded.

Cancellous screws can be fully or partly threaded, and are designed for use in the loose cancellous or spongy bone found in the heads of long bones. These have more widely spaced threads than the cortical screws and narrower shafts.

Both cortical and cancellous screws have a hex screwdriver fitting.

21. D *Jacob's chuck is used to position intramedullary pins*

22. C *The needle holders that have scissors combined are the Olsen–Hegar needle holders*

23. C *The pilot hole for a 3.5-mm ASIF cortical screw should be drilled using a 2.5 mm drill bit*
The quoted diameter of a screw is diameter of the widest part of the thread. If a 3.5 mm hole was drilled, a 3.5-mm screw would simply drop through without biting.

24. A *The forceps that have a rat tooth end are Lane's forceps*
Lane's forceps are one of the most commonly used types of tissue forceps.
   Spey forceps and Bendover forceps are atraumatic dressing forceps with plain ends.
   Allis tissue forceps are self-retaining forceps with a ratchet, used for retracting tissue. They have small serrations on the jaws to help grip, but are not as severe as the rat tooth end.

25. C *Instruments should be passed to a surgeon with the ratchet closed, rings first*

26. C *Strabismus scissors are used for ophthalmic surgery*
These are small, delicate scissors used for fine surgery of the eye.

27. A *Halstead mosquito forceps are used as a haemostat*
Allis tissue forceps are used for holding tissues out of the surgical field.
   Adson dissecting forceps are another type of rat tooth forceps used for general surgery.
   Cheatle forceps are used by a non-sterile person to transfer sterile items from one place to another.

28. C *The No. 11 blade is known as a tenotomy blade*
This is a fine-pointed blade, which can be used for splitting tendons.

29. D *Temperatures as low as −150°C can be reached using liquid nitrogen for cryotherapy*
This is the temperature that can be reached using liquid nitrogen with a probe. Using the liquid nitrogen as a spray, even lower temperatures (down to −196°C) can be achieved. Gaseous nitrous oxide can also be used as a cryogen, but temperatures only reach −50°C with this.

21 Fluid therapy and shock

1. B *The dog requires 1000 ml for rehydration*
If the dog is 8% dehydrated, it has lost 8% of its body weight.
Calculate 8% of the body weight:
  $= 8/100 \times 12.5\,\text{kg}$
  $= 1\,\text{kg}$
This is the weight of the fluid that has been lost.
1 litre of water weighs 1 kg, therefore this dog has lost 1 litre of fluid.
1 l = 1000 ml, therefore the fluid deficit for this dog is 1000 ml.

2. D *The fluid that should be used intravenously to maintain an animal once it is rehydrated is 0.18% sodium chloride, 4% dextrose ($\frac{1}{5}$ normal saline)*

3. B *The drip should be set to provide one drop every 2 seconds*
You need to give 2160 ml in 24 hours.
Therefore, you need to give 2160/24 ml in 1 hour
  $= 90\,\text{ml/hour, or } 90/60\,\text{ml/min}$
  $= 1.5\,\text{ml/min}$
If 1 ml/min $= 20$ drops, then 1.5 ml/min
    $= 1.5 \times 20\,\text{drops/min}$
    $= 30\,\text{drops/min, or } 30/60\,\text{drops/sec}$
    $= 0.5\,\text{drops/sec, or 1 drop every 2 seconds.}$

4. A *Sodium bicarbonate should not be given with Hartmann's solution*
Hartmann's solution contains calcium ions. If sodium bicarbonate were added to Hartmann's solution it would react with the calcium to produce solid calcium carbonate, which would precipitate out within the drip. Ringer's solution also contains calcium ions, so sodium bicarbonate should not be used with this either.
  Sodium bicarbonate is used in cases of severe acidosis to absorb excess hydrogen ions within the body, and can be given with normal saline, 5% dextrose, or 0.18% sodium chloride in 4% dextrose.

5. B *Over-infusion of intravenous fluids could lead to the development of oedema*
If over-infusion of intravenous fluid occurs, the circulation becomes overloaded and blood pressure increases. This forces fluid out of capillaries into the interstitial spaces, and this is

evident as oedema. The site of oedema development depends on the type of fluid being infused. Colloids remain in the circulation, which increases the workload of the heart. Eventually the heart is unable to cope and blood dams back into the systemic circulation, leading to oedema and ascites due to right-sided congestive heart failure.

Crystalloids do not remain in the circulation, but equilibrate throughout all the fluid compartments. Therefore the whole body becomes saturated with fluid, and oedema forms in all tissues.

6. C *Plasma forms approximately 5% of an animal's total body weight*
The total fluid within the body accounts for between 60 and 70% of an animal's body weight. This is divided into intracellular fluid (40–50% of body weight) and extracellular fluid (20% of body weight). The ECF is divided further into the interstitial fluid (15% of body weight), plasma and lymph (5% of body weight), and the transcellular fluids (< 1% of body weight). Synovial fluid forms a small fraction of the transcellular fluids.

7. A *Unconsciousness results in a primary water deficit*
A primary water deficit occurs when there is loss of fluid from the body without electrolyte losses. This can arise in any situation where either the animal is unable to drink or where insensible losses through respiration and sweat are increased. Possible causes therefore include water deprivation, unconsciousness and heat stroke.

Vomiting, diarrhoea and burns all result in dehydration with the loss of electrolytes as well as water.

8. A *The anticoagulant that is used when collecting blood for blood transfusions is acid citrate dextrose*
Heparin is the anticoagulant used for biochemical studies. EDTA is used for haematology, and fluoride oxalate prevents clotting in samples for glucose assessment.

9. A *Normal central venous pressure in small animals is 3–7 cm H_2O*
Central venous pressure can be measured using a jugular catheter attached to a giving set, a three-way tap and a water manometer.

Arterial pressure is far higher than venous pressure, and is measured in millimetres of mercury (mm Hg). Normal arterial pressures for cats and dogs are about 150–160 mm Hg.

10. D *1.8% sodium chloride is not isotonic*
Almost all the crystalloid fluids routinely used in veterinary practice are isotonic. This means that they exert the same osmotic pressure as fluid within cells, so giving these intravenously does not cause water to move into or out of the cells through osmosis.

11. C *Hartmann's solution would be the most suitable to use to rehydrate an animal with chronic diarrhoea*
An animal suffering from chronic diarrhoea would have lost a considerable amount of water, and would also have lost many electrolytes from the intestinal secretions. The most important of these are sodium and bicarbonate. Hartmann's solution contains sodium, calcium and lactate. It does not contain bicarbonate, because the calcium would precipitate out as calcium carbonate. However, the lactate is metabolized into bicarbonate within the body.

12. D *The cat requires 280 ml of fluid*
For every 1% increase in packed cell volume (PCV), the animal has lost 10 ml/kg.
Therefore, calculate the increase in PCV:
$$44 - 37 = 7\%$$
Then calculate the deficit per kg:
$$7 \times 10\,\text{ml/kg} = 70\,\text{ml/kg}$$
Then calculate the total deficit:
$$70 \times 4 = 280\,\text{ml}$$

13. A *Potassium might need to be supplemented in the drip of an anorexic cat being maintained on intravenous fluids*
Animals which are not eating or which have been starved will be deficient in many electrolytes, including sodium and potassium. The hormone aldosterone, produced by the adrenal cortex, is responsible for maintaining sodium levels within the body, and is released if sodium concentrations fall. It acts on the renal tubules to conserve sodium and to excrete potassium ions in exchange.

However, potassium is essential for normal fluid balance within the body and for normal nerve and muscle function, and without it cardiac dysrrhythmias and muscle weakness can develop. Animals that are being given prolonged fluid therapy should therefore be given additional potassium.

14. C *Shock does not cause a marked parasympathetic response*
Shock is a condition in which there is progressive deterioration of the circulation, so that there is decreased delivery of oxygen to the tissues. It is an emergency situation, since without treatment the vital organs become so hypoxic that they are unable to function adequately and death follows. Shock can be caused by anything that seriously affects the circulation, and is categorized into three types: hypovolaemic shock, caused by blood loss or dehydration; maldistributive shock or vasculogenic shock, caused by severe vasodilation, which results in a fall in blood pressure and failure of tissue perfusion; and cardiogenic shock, caused by heart failure, which is rare in small animals.

22 Anaesthesia and analgesia

1. B *The premedication agent that has significant analgesic effects is buprenorphine*

Buprenorphine is an opiate that produces good analgesia and some central nervous system depression.

Acepromazine produces mental calmness at low doses, but is a sedative at higher doses. Atropine is used for its effects in countering the production of saliva in the anaesthetized patient.

Diazepam is a tranquillizer. It is particularly useful in older patients, as it has minimal respiratory or cardiovascular effects.

2. C *A 50 kg animal will require 1 ml*

First calculate the dose needed:

Dose = dose rate × body weight

$\qquad$ = 0.006 × 50 mg

$\qquad$ = 0.3 mg

Then calculate the volume needed:

$\quad$ Volume = dose/concentration

$\qquad\qquad$ = 0.3/0.3 ml

$\qquad\qquad$ = 1 ml

3. D *The problems associated with the use of small animal Immobilon include cyanosis, hypotension and bradycardia in the patient, and the risk of accidental self-administration by the operator*

Small animal Immobilon contains two components: etorphine, an opiate, and methotrimeprazine, a sedative. Immobilon is an extremely dangerous drug, and should only be used in the presence of someone who is able to give the antidote in case of accidental self-administration. For humans the antidote is naloxone (Narcan), which reverses the opiate part of the combination although the sedative effects persist.

The drug produces excellent analgesia in the patient, but the anaesthesia is difficult to control with the patient often developing severe hypotension and cyanosis. Relaxation can be variable, and there have been accounts of renal failure developing after its use. There are many better and safer products available nowadays.

4. C *The Magill is classified as a semi-closed circuit*
There are four categories of anaesthetic circuits:

The open circuit consists of nothing more than an anaesthetic-soaked gauze held up to the patient's nose. This is sometimes referred to as the 'rag and bottle' method.

The semi-open circuit is a similar arrangement, with a gauze pad soaked in anaesthetic, except that there is a head collar or other device that prevents the animal from breathing around the pad.

The semi-closed method includes the majority of anaesthetic circuits, such as the Magill, T-piece, Lack and Bain. The patient is given a controlled gas supply that contains a specific amount of anaesthetic agent, and exhaled gases are vented away from the animal.

A closed circuit is one in which the patient rebreathes exhaled gases after the removal of carbon dioxide. This is usually achieved through the use of a soda-lime canister. Examples of this type of circuit include the to and fro circuit, or the Circle system.

Note: If American text books are referred to, the classification system is different in the States to that used in the UK.

5. B *Recovery from thiopentone-induced anaesthesia takes place through initial redistribution of the thiopentone to fatty tissues, and then gradual metabolism by the liver*
Thiopentone is very lipid soluble and, after affecting the brain to produce anaesthesia, is redistributed through all the fatty tissues of the body. As a result, the concentration in the brain falls and the animal wakes up. However, there is still thiopentone within the body tissues, and this is then metabolized and removed by the liver over a much longer period of time.

Thin animals have little body fat, so the thiopentone remains within the central nervous system tissue for longer and recovery is prolonged.

6. C *Alphaxalone and alphadolone acetate must not be given to dogs*
This mixture, marketed as Saffan, must not be used in dogs because they can develop anaphylactic reactions to the 20% cremophor solution used as the carrier for the steroids.

Ketamine can be used in dogs, but only in combination with other drugs such as xylazine (Rompun) or diazepam (Valium), or it can induce fits.

Propofol (Rapinovet) and methohexitone sodium (Brietal) can be used safely as anaesthetic agents in dogs.

7. C *Buprenorphine is controlled under Schedule 3 of The Misuse of Drugs Act 1971*
The Misuse of Drugs Act 1971 and the Misuse of Drugs Regulations 1985 were introduced in order to control the use of drugs that were considered to have the potential to be drugs of abuse. It divides the different products into five Schedules according to the risk. Schedule 1 contains products such as cannabis and LSD, which are considered to have no therapeutic uses, but are addictive. Schedule 2 contains most of the opiates, including morphine and pethidine. Schedule 3 contains buprenorphine, as it is considered to have a lower abuse potential than the other opiates. This schedule also includes the barbiturates, such as phenobarbitone.

Diazepam and butorphanol are included in Schedule 4 with some other sedatives and anabolic steroids, and Schedule 5 products are those that only contain very small quantities of drugs listed in the higher schedules.

8. D *Trichloroethylene must not be used with soda-lime*
If trichloroethylene and soda-lime are mixed, several noxious products are produced, including phosgene and hydrochloric acid. Trichloroethylene is usually coloured with a blue dye as a warning to prevent this occurring.

9. B *The pressure in a nitrous oxide tank decreases when all of the liquid nitrous oxide has vaporized and the tank is almost empty*
Pressure gauges on cylinders that contain gases in a liquid form cannot be used as a means of estimating the quantity of agent remaining, as the pressure gauge only indicates the pressure of the gas above the liquid. This stays constant until there is no liquid remaining. The only way to tell how much gas is left is to weigh the cylinder and compare it with the weights of full and empty cylinders. The empty cylinder weight (or tare) is stamped on the side of the cylinder valve block.

10. B *Anticholinergics may be included in premedication for cats and dogs to decrease saliva and bronchial secretions*
The anticholinergics antagonize the effects of the parasympathetic nervous system, and decrease the unwanted autonomic effects produced by these neurones. The anticholinergics also have other effects that are not necessarily beneficial, such as increasing the heart rate and producing pupil dilation, and for this reason they are now less widely used than previously. The most commonly used drug of this type is atropine sulphate.

11. A *Pethidine is a narcotic*
The term 'narcotic' is used to describe drugs that are derived from opium. Narcotics include pethidine, morphine, buprenorphine, butorphanol and codeine.

Xylazine (Rompun) and medetomidine (Domitor) are both examples of α_2-agonists, which produce marked sedation.

Ketamine is a cyclohexanone, and is sometimes described as a dissociative anaesthetic because of the effect it produces in man.

Propofol is a water-soluble phenol, which produces both rapid induction and recovery from anaesthesia.

12. C *Ketamine does not produce a fall in blood pressure*
Ketamine causes an increase in heart rate, so the blood pressure remains normal or may even be increased. Ketamine also causes increased muscle tone and muscle twitching, and should not be used on its own in the dog.

Xylazine and medetomidine produce a transient increase in blood pressure before causing a marked hypotension.

Acepromazine also produces hypotension, especially when high dose rates are used.

13. D *Xylazine and medetomidine produce all the effects listed*
Despite these disadvantages, medetomidine (Domitor) and xylazine (Rompun) are widely used since they produce good relaxation and a good degree of analgesia. Medetomidine also has the advantage of having a reversal agent, atipamezole (Antisedan).

14. A *A size E oxygen cylinder contains 680 litres*

15. C *An analeptic is a drug that stimulates the central nervous system*
Analeptics are drugs that stimulate the central nervous system, and include doxapram (Dopram), which is used to stimulate the respiratory centre within the brain.

Drugs that cause drowsiness are described as sedatives.

Ataractics produce calmness without drowsiness, for example acepromazine (at low doses) or the benzodiazepines.

Drugs that decrease the sensation of pain are analgesics.

16. A *Methohexitone sodium is an example of a barbiturate anaesthetic*
Methohexitone sodium (Brietal) is a barbiturate that is more rapidly metabolized by the liver than thiopentone, and so is more suitable for use in lean animals.

Alphaxalone and alphadolone (Saffan) are steroids. Ketamine is a cyclohexanone, and propofol is a phenol.

17. D *A neuro-leptanaesthetic is a mixture of a sedative with an opioid analgesic*
Neuro-leptanaesthetics are drug combinations that can be used in a variety of species. Small and large animal Immobilon and Hypnorm are examples of drugs used for this type of anaesthesia. They produce marked respiratory and cardiovascular depression, and variable muscle relaxation. Often the animals still remain sensitive to external stimuli such as sound.

18. A *Methoxyflurane has the lowest MAC number*
MAC is an abbreviation for minimum alveolar concentration, and MAC numbers are used as a means of describing the potency of an anaesthetic. The minimum alveolar concentration is a measurement of the concentration of an anaesthetic agent within the alveoli that is needed to prevent a response to a particular stimulus. The concentration is expressed as a percentage. Anaesthetics with low MAC numbers are therefore more potent than those with high numbers.

Methoxyflurane has a MAC number of 0.23, halothane 0.8, nitrous oxide 188–220, and isoflurane 1.3.

Nitrous oxide has a MAC number of over 100 because it is impossible to give sufficient agent on its own to prevent a response to the particular stimulus. It only has weak anaesthetic properties. However, it is useful in combination with other anaesthetic agents to improve analgesia.

19. B *The combination usually used is 2 : 1 nitrous oxide : oxygen*
Nitrous oxide is often used with oxygen as a carrier gas in inhalation anaesthesia. It has weak anaesthetic and analgesic properties, which means that the dose of volatile anaesthetic agent required can be reduced.

It is very readily taken up by haemoglobin within blood cells, even more so than oxygen, so it should never exceed 80% of the gas mixture or hypoxia could arise. At the end of anaesthesia, the nitrous oxide should be turned off and pure oxygen administered for at least 3 minutes. This is to allow the nitrous oxide to be exhaled before the animal starts to breathe air, which only contains about 20% oxygen.

Nitrous oxide should not be used if there is a gas-filled area within the animal's body, such as a gastric dilation or pneumothorax. Nitrous oxide readily diffuses into these areas, and compromises the animal by increasing the pressure within the tissues.

20. C *The anaesthetic used by Guedel to classify the stages of anaesthesia was ether*
Most of Guedel's observations are still true for the modern anaesthetics, although stages I and II, the induction stages, are passed through quickly and are not very obvious with intravenous agents.

21. A *The Lack circuit requires the use of 1–1.5 × minute volume*
To prevent the patient rebreathing, semi-closed anaesthetic circuits require a minimum fresh gas flow rate. The Lack and Magill need 1–1.5 × minute volume (the amount of air an animal breathes in and out in one minute). The Ayre's T-piece and the Bain use higher fresh gas flow rates, 2.5–3 × minute volume.

The minute volume is often estimated as 200 ml/kg, although this will vary considerably for individual animals depending on age and disease conditions, respiratory rate and the procedure for which the animal is being anaesthetized.

22. C *Silicates are included in soda-lime to prevent it from forming an irritant dust*
Soda-lime consists mainly of calcium hydroxide and sodium hydroxide. These compounds are quite alkaline, and if allowed to crumble will produce significant irritation of the patient's airway.

The hydroxides remove exhaled carbon dioxide by reacting with it and moisture to produce carbonates.

23. B *Suxamethonium is a depolarizing neuromuscular blocker*
Neuromuscular blockers or muscle relaxants prevent nervous
impulses from reaching skeletal muscles and produce
paralysis. There are two types of blockers: depolarizing
blockers such as suxamethonium, and non-depolarizing
blockers such as vecuronium, gallamine, atracuronium and
pancuronium.

Non-depolarizing drugs are reversed by neostigmine. There is
no true antidote for the depolarizing blockers, but neostigmine
partially reverses their effects. Neostigmine should always be
used with an anticholinergic such as atropine.

24. C *As an animal becomes anaesthetized, the first reflex to be lost is
the swallowing reflex*
The swallowing reflex is lost quite early in anaesthesia. Once it
has been lost, the airway is usually protected by the use of
endotracheal tubes with inflatable cuffs which prevent any
secretions or vomit entering the trachea while the animal is
unconscious. Endotracheal tubes should only be removed once
the swallowing reflex starts to return.

The pedal reflex, anal reflex and palpebral reflexes can all be
used during anaesthesia to determine whether the patient is
under light, medium or deep surgical anaesthesia.

25. C *According to the Health and Safety Executive, the maximum
length of tubing suitable for use with a passive scavenging
system is 8.5 ft or 2.6 m*
Passive scavenging relies on the gas flow from the anaesthetic
machine and the patient exhaling to drive the contaminated gas
through the ducting and out of the theatre. If the tubing is too
long, the gases will pool within the piping and re-enter the
operating theatre once surgery finishes. It also means that the
resistance against which the patient has to breathe is quite
high.

26. B *The anaesthetic gas supplied in blue cylinders is nitrous oxide*
All the anaesthetic gases are supplied in colour-coded
cylinders. Oxygen comes in black cylinders with a white neck,
carbon dioxide is supplied in grey cylinders, and
cyclopropane is found in orange cylinders.

27. B *Activated charcoal within a circuit removes halothane*
In some passive scavenging systems, adsorbers containing activated charcoal are used. These only remove halothane. If nitrous oxide is being used, this still constitutes a potential hazard for the operators.

Soda-lime removes carbon dioxide, but does not affect either nitrous oxide or halothane concentrations.

28. B *You would need to draw up 0.02 ml of thiopentone for the mouse*
This calculation needs to be carried out in three stages.
First, calculate the dose of agent needed by the mouse:
Dose = dose rate × body weight
Convert the mouse weight into kg:
Weight in kg = 50/1000 kg
= 0.05 kg
Therefore, dose = 10 × 0.05
= 0.5 mg
Secondly, convert the concentration of the thiopentone from % into mg/ml:
2.5% = 2.5 g in 100 ml, or 2.5 × 1000 mg in 100 ml
= 2500 mg in 100 ml
= 25 mg in 1 ml, or 25 mg/ml
Finally, calculate the volume needed:
Volume = dose/concentration
= 0.5/25 ml
= 0.02 ml

29. A *The intravenous anaesthetic with the shortest recovery time is propofol*
If propofol (Rapinovet) is given as a single bolus, it is very quickly metabolized by the liver and the animal recovers rapidly.

Methohexitone sodium is also broken down by the liver fairly rapidly.

30. C *Under Guedel's classification, surgical anaesthesia is Stage III*
Guedel used ether on human patients to classify the stages of anaesthesia:
Stage I is the stage of voluntary excitement.
Stage II is the stage of involuntary excitement. Stages I and II are passed through during induction of anaesthesia.
Stage III is surgical anaesthesia and is divided into three planes; plane 1 is light, plane 2 is medium and plane 3 is deep anaesthesia.
Stage IV is the stage of overdosage.

31. A *Muscle relaxants act at the neuromuscular junction*

32. D *The flow rate suitable for the cat on a T-piece is 2000 ml/min*
To calculate the fresh gas flow rate for a patient, you first need to estimate the animal's minute volume. If the respiration rate is not given, then a general allowance for the minute volume is made – approximately 200 ml/kg.
Therefore for this cat, the minute volume
$$= 200 \times 4 = 800\,\text{ml/min}$$
An allowance then has to be made for the specific circuit being used. In this case the T-piece was in use, which requires a fresh gas flow rate of 2.5–3 × minute volume.
Therefore, the fresh gas flow rate $= 2.5$–$3 \times 800\,\text{ml/min}$
$$= 2000\text{–}2400\,\text{ml/min},$$
and the suggested answer of 2000 ml/min would therefore be appropriate.

23 Radiography

1. D *The grid factor for a grid depends on the grid ratio, the lines per centimetre and the thickness of the lines*
The grid factor is the number by which the mAs has to be multiplied when using the grid in order to give the same radiographic density as if the grid was not present.

2. D *The technique would be described as retrograde urethrography*
Intravenous urography is a technique used to highlight the kidneys and ureters by giving a water-soluble contrast medium intravenously. For showing up the kidneys a bolus is usually used, whereas for the ureters a slow infusion produces better results.

Positive contrast cystography would be performed in a similar way to retrograde urethrography, except that the contrast medium would be delivered specifically to the bladder rather than just into the urethra.

3. B *The new exposure factors are FFD = 70 cm, kV = 45 kV, mA = 15 mA*
In every calculation regarding exposure factors, the mAs should be calculated first. This gives an indication of the number of X-rays reaching the film.
mAs = 20 × 0.3 = 6 mAs
If the time or the mA have to be changed, the mAs should always remain the same to maintain the same radiographic density. Therefore:
New mA × new time = 6 mAs
New mA × 0.4 = 6 mAs
To determine the New mA, divide both sides by 0.4:
New mA = 6/0.4 = 15 mA

4. C *The radiation-sensitive grains are found in the emulsion layer of the X-ray film*
The supercoat is a protective layer that overlies the emulsion.

The subbing layer sticks the emulsion to the polyester base that provides the support for the emulsion.

5. D *Altering the kV will affect the quality of the X-ray beam*
The quality of the X-ray beam is related to the energy of the X-ray photons within the beam. This is controlled by changing the kV, which alters the potential difference between the

cathode and the anode. If the difference between the cathode and anode is increased, the electrons will travel faster across the vacuum and the X-rays produced will have higher energy.

The mA controls the current through the wire filament, which results in the release of the electrons. Increasing the current means more electrons are available to move across the tube head, and so more X-rays will be produced. Similarly, increasing the time means that the potential difference is applied for longer and more electrons have time to cross from the cathode to the anode, so more X-rays will be produced.

Changing the focal–film distance alters the density of the final radiograph. If the distance is increased, then the energy of the X-rays reaching the plate is the same and the number of X-rays is the same, but they are spread over a wider area.

6. **D** *The absorption of X-rays by a tissue depends on its atomic number, the density and the thickness of the tissue.*
The absorption of X-rays depends on all three factors. Therefore bone, which is very dense, and iodine, which has a high atomic number, are radiopaque and show up white on radiographs. Conversely, gas, which has a relatively low atomic number and is not dense, is easily penetrated by X-rays and shows up black on radiographs.

7. **D** *Unexposed silver bromide grains are washed off the film in the fixer*
During processing, the developer converts exposed silver bromide grains into black metallic silver. The fixer removes any unexposed silver bromide to leave the final image.

8. **C** *Low osmolar, non-ionic water-soluble iodine preparations should be used as contrast media for myelograms*
These materials are the most inert of all the contrast media, and therefore produce the least damage to the central nervous system and the least side effects.

The high osmolar water-soluble iodine-containing compounds can be used for intravascular contrast studies and for examination of the upper urinary tract, since they are excreted by the kidneys.

Barium compounds are usually used for gastro-intestinal contrast studies, and are either given orally or per rectum.

9. C *The greatest amount of radiation a person may legally be exposed to in a year is the maximum permissible dose*
The maximum permissible doses (MPDs) are arbitrary doses thought not to carry a significant health risk. Members of the public, including veterinary nurses, should receive less than these doses in a year. Designated workers, such as those dealing with larger radiation sources, have a different set of MPDs. The figures are for adults over 18 years old. People under 16 should receive no dose at all, and those between the ages of 16 and 18 have intermediate MPDs.

10. D *The use of X-rays in practice is controlled by The Ionising Radiations Regulations 1999*
The Ionising Radiations Regulations 1999 is a very complex piece of legislation, so Guidance Notes for the Protection of Persons against Ionising Radiations arising from Veterinary Use were drawn up. This is not a piece of legislation, but an explanation of the law as it applies to veterinary practices.

11. B *A film that had been overexposed would have a black background, and the subject would also be too dark*
Overexposure means that either too many X-rays have reached the plate, or the X-rays had too much energy and so were able to pass through the subject too easily. The exposure factors should be reduced to correct this fault.
A film in which the background is black but the subject is white has been underexposed. In most cases this means that the X-rays lacked sufficient energy to pass through the tissues, and the kV should be increased to rectify the problem.
If a film has a grey background and it is possible to see a finger held up behind it, this is suggestive of underdevelopment. It could be that the film was not developed for long enough, that the developer chemical was becoming exhausted, or that the temperature of the developer was too cold.
Finally, if one area of the radiograph is black, it could be because the film has been exposed to light in some way. The box of film could have been left open, or the cassette might not have been closed properly.

12. C *If the distance between the effective focal spot and the film is trebled, then the mAs should be increased by nine times to maintain the same radiographic density*
As the focal–film distance is increased, the area over which the X-rays are spread becomes greater. The Inverse Square Law

states this mathematically: 'the intensity of the X-ray beam is inversely proportional to the focal–film distance squared'.

To compensate for the decrease in intensity, the mAs has to be increased. If the distance is trebled, the mAs has to be increased by a factor of 3 squared, i.e. 9.

13. D *X-rays are not reflected by any materials*
They are not reflected, but are able to penetrate all materials to some degree. X-rays travel in straight lines, and will affect photographic emulsion such that it appears black after processing.

14. B *Parallel grids can result in grid cut-off at the edge of the radiograph*
The primary beam is not a parallel beam, but diverges towards the edge of the area being radiographed. Angled X-ray photons at the edge are unable to pass between the vertical slats of a parallel grid, and so fewer X-rays reach the plate. This phenomenon is called grid cut-off.

Pseudo-focused and focused grids are designed to compensate for this. However, these grids are not identical. Focused grids have slats that are progressively sloped at the same angle as the X-rays within the primary beam, so that they are vertical in the centre but become more angled towards the edge of the grid. Pseudo-focused grids have vertical lead slats that get shorter and shorter towards the edge of the grid, so that the angled X-ray photons can pass between them and reach the plate.

The Potter Bucky grid is a moving grid. It moves very rapidly backwards and forwards during the exposure so that grid lines are not visible on the final radiograph.

Regardless of the type of grid being used, the exposure factors have to be increased because some of the primary beam X-rays are absorbed as well as scattered X-rays.

15. C *Heat is lost by radiation through the vacuum in the rotating anode X-ray tube head*
In the stationary anode tube head, heat is lost from the target by conduction through a copper rod to the oil bath. This method cannot be used in the rotating anode tube head, because it would conduct the heat to the motor and damage it. Radiation is therefore the only means by which the heat can be lost.

Convection and evaporation are impossible because there is no medium within the tube head, just a vacuum.

16. C *The step-up transformer is needed to increase the voltage*
between the anode and cathode from 240 V to 40–80 kV

There is a rectifier in the tube head, which changes alternating
current into direct current, and a step-down transformer changes
the mains voltage to 10 V.

There is also an autotransformer within the tube head, which
smooths out fluctuations in the mains voltage so that
radiographic quality is consistent.

17. C *Non-screen film should be left in the developer 1 minute longer*
than screen film, if being processed manually at 20°C

18. C *The settings kV = 80 kV, mA = 40 mA, time = 0.2 secs,*
FFD = 70 cm could be used
First calculate the original mAs:
Original mAs = $20 \times 0.2 = 4$ mAs

Then introduce the grid factor 4 to give the new mAs:
New mAs = 4×4
$= 16$ mAs

Then check the answers you have been given to see if any of
them give an mAs of 16, without changing any of the
exposure factors other than the time and the mA.

In this example there are no answers that fit.

There is, however, a rule of thumb that can be applied if the
mAs becomes too high. Increasing the kV by 10 means that the
mAs can be halved, and this will result in radiographs of the
same appearance.

Therefore, if the kV is increased to 80 kV, the mAs can be
reduced to 8 mAs.

Now check the possible answers for one with these factors.

19. B *The radius of the controlled area from the X-ray tube head*
when used in an unconfined area is 2 m

20. A *Computed tomography, or CT scanning, uses an X-ray tube*
head to generate its images
CT scanning produces a very detailed radiograph of a thin
cross-section through the animal's tissues. Many radiographs
are taken, each in a slightly different position, so large
doses of radiation are used and the animals need to be
anaesthetized.

Magnetic resonance imaging (MRI scanning) uses magnetism and radio waves to generate the images, whereas ultrasound uses very high frequency sound waves that are not detectable with the ear. Scintigraphy does involve the use of radiation, but it is administered to the patient in the form of radioactive chemicals given intravenously.

21. C *Grids cannot be used to decrease the production of scattered radiation*
In fact, grids result in more scatter being produced, because the exposure factors have to be increased to compensate for their use. What the grids do is prevent the final image being disrupted by the effects of scattered radiation reaching the film.

Compressing the part being radiographed decreases the thickness of the tissue, and so will cut down the scatter produced. However, this technique is not often used as it could compromise or harm the patient in some way, or it is impossible because the tissue being radiographed is bony.

Collimating tightly reduces scatter by limiting the radiation to just the amount needed to produce a diagnostic film. The use of lead-backed cassettes helps by reducing backscatter.

22. B *The use of screens does not mean that higher exposure factors are required than without screens*
Screens contain crystals that fluoresce when exposed to radiation. X-ray film is both light- and radiation-sensitive, so this means that a single X-ray photon passing through the screens and film will cause both a direct effect on the film, and an indirect effect due to the light from the fluorescent crystals within the screens. The screens therefore amplify the effect of the radiation, and so reduce the number of X-rays needed.

The light produced by the crystals spreads for a short distance in all directions, so that the use of screens does decrease the definition of the radiograph slightly.

23. B *The aluminium filter in the window of the X-ray tube head absorbs any low energy X-rays*
When X-rays are produced most have the same energy, but there are also some with lower energies. These would be too weak to be of any diagnostic value but would still contribute to the biological hazard to the patient and operators, so they are removed by an aluminium filter which is placed over the window through which the primary beam passes.

24. C *Developer solutions should be kept in a tank with the lid on to prevent oxidation of the chemicals*
As the chemicals are oxidized they become exhausted, so by keeping the lid on the useful life span of a solution is increased.